THE SMART GIRL'S HANDBOOK TO BEING

Mummylicious

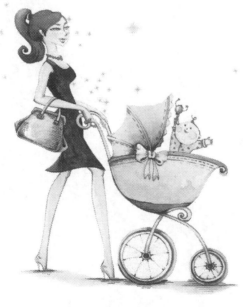

CHRISTINE AMOUR-LEVAR

www.thesmartgirlshandbook.com

THE SMART GIRL'S HANDBOOK TO BEING

Mummylicious

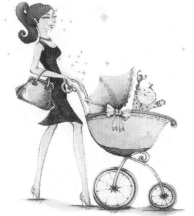

Written by:
CHRISTINE AMOUR-LEVAR

Illustrated by :
WEARN

Designed by :
NATHALIE HUNI

Edited by :
REINE MARIE MELVIN & GISELLE GO

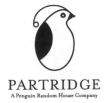

PARTRIDGE

A Penguin Random House Company

To order additional copies of this book, contact
Toll Free 800 101 2657 (Singapore)
Toll Free 1 800 81 7340 (Malaysia)
orders.singapore@partridgepublishing.com

www.partridgepublishing.com/singapore

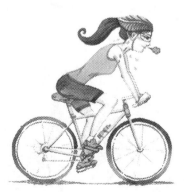

Contents

To my beautiful children,
Yasmine, Malcolm, Louis and Angeline,
without whom I could never have written this book.
Know that I love you and that I am forever
grateful for you in my life.

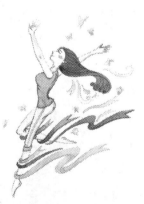

Foreword
by Kristin Armstrong Eberstadt

I believe that every mother, secretly or not, wants to be **Mummylicious** - the best version of herself in body, mind, and spirit after a pregnancy. Yes, even you. That's why you picked up this book. But, like me and many other women, you make excuses: "it's too hard","I'm too busy", "my children need me, my husband needs me, my boss needs me, my dog needs me", "it's selfish", "it's vain", "I'll focus on myself when the kids are in college", "my body has just changed and it can never be the same again, so pass the cake", "I deserve that cake!" STOP. Just stop. This book will help you quiet the noises in your head, and inspire you to stop making excuses and start becoming the woman you know you are and can be.

Reading this book is like sitting with the kind of girlfriend you always wanted. The kind of friend who tells you the truth (even if it hurts just a little at first), because she cares about you deeply and knows your potential. She'll tell you getting back into shape after a pregnancy is hard work, but she'll give you the tools to get there. She won't abandon you after that either, but continue to motivate you and challenge you. She'll tell you not to give up that job, that hobby, or that dream either. Her voice will stay with you, when those other voices take over "I'll never change", "my dreams can wait", "I can't do it", "Who cares? No one is looking at me anyway", "the baby is the only thing I should worry about now", "pass that cake already!"

I was fortunate to have that girlfriend long before this book was written. The author and I have been friends since college. I have watched her live this book, and all the tips in it. I've seen it work. I'll never forget watching her hand over her first newborn daughter to her mother, so that she could go to the gym for 20 minutes. When I had my newborn, I could barely get out of my pajamas, let alone think about going to the gym. Again those voices in my head. I get it, the constant juggling you, as a mother, have to do, between your children, spouse, house, job, whatever. Inevitably, there is not much time left for you. Here's the secret: you can have it all! Christine will show you how and be with you every step of the way with concrete steps that really work. You can be **Mummylicious** too. Just do it.

Start today. I'll let you sit with a good girlfriend for a while…

Introduction
Why I Wrote this Book

I remember clearly a day when I was 10 years old, sitting around a country club pool surrounded by my mother's friends and their children happily splashing about. Most of these mothers were in their mid-to late thirties, with sizeable bottoms and generous waistlines, while the few fathers who were there that day sported rounded beer guts and love handles to match.

On the far side of the pool area, another mother arrived with her three young children in tow. She was wearing an elegant white bikini on her trim athletic frame, and as she set about arranging her things and her children around her by the pool, the mindless chatter stopped abruptly, and the envious and awed staring began. Even I, in my prepubescent state, quickly realized that this woman was an exception. She had a confidence to her stride that other mothers didn't seem to have. She was in no way a classic beauty, but there emanated from her poise, a quiet and elegant sexiness and self-assurance that was hard to ignore. Even at 10 years of age, the image of this attractive and elegant-looking young mother entered my consciousness, and I asked myself there and then: "When I have children of my own one day, why can't I be that kind of woman?" This realisation stayed with me for the rest of my life.

Today I have been blessed with four beautiful children. I gained about 17 kilos (or 37 pounds) for each pregnancy. My babies were not that large despite this very respectable weight gain; they were on average about three kilos (or seven pounds) each. After each delivery, I found myself with a good 12 to 14 kilos (26 to 30 pounds) to shed, which is quite sizable on my average frame. After every single one of these four pregnancies, I found the discipline and the willpower to re-conquer my figure - fighting every inch of fat and flab of the way back to my original weight and size. It was no easy achievement.

I wrote this book because I wanted to share with other mothers the physical and mental tools that helped me get my body and my groove back after each of these four grueling pregnancies. No matter how much weight a girl puts on during pregnancy, be it 10 or 30 kilos or more, my tried and proven solution can get you back to your dream weight if you are committed to giving it your complete and unwavering dedication. Without claiming to be a fitness expert or a nutritionist, I did my research and tried numerous methods in depth and have found an ideal process that has rewarded me with continued and lasting success.

The sense of achievement and pride that comes with regaining your pre-pregnancy figure and weight cannot be underestimated. It gives a woman that extra dose of confidence that arms her for success in whatever she chooses to do in her life. It shows she cares enough about herself to take the time and energy to look her best, and it's visual proof that she can achieve anything she sets her mind to.

Getting your figure back is just the beginning. It opens up countless opportunities for you to grow in confidence and positivity. The ultimate objective is not simply to look great and be healthy, but also to feel truly fulfilled in your life as a woman and as a new mother. Nevertheless, let me tell you right now that if you hope to miraculously get back into your jeans two weeks after giving birth like one of these supermodel mums we've all seen on TV, then this book is not for you. This book is for the rest of us women who need to work hard to get back into shape after having a baby. This is for the kind of woman who knows deep inside that she has to give something to get something in return, and who is committed to being disciplined in order to achieve that goal for herself and her body. That body has been stretched beyond recognition, endured over nine months of hormonal changes, endless cravings, cramps, water retention, swelling, nausea, poor sleep – and has also been the home of a little kicking and wiggling alien for these long months. That body needs healing, care and strengthening after each pregnancy, until it really begins to feel like your own again. And the day will come when you will be able to slip on that sexy cocktail dress you used to wear, which has been hanging in your closet accumulating dust for the past year and a half or more. That's when you'll know that you've finally got your body and your groove back - and that you've earned it every inch of the way!

What Does it Mean
to be MUMMYLICIOUS?

Being **Mummylicious** means being the best and most attractive you can possibly be as a woman and as a mother. A woman who is **Mummylicious** oozes confidence and femininity and defies the conventional image we have of frumpy motherhood. She is committed to taking care of herself, body and mind, and always tries to look and be at her best. She is first and foremost a woman – not just a mother.

But being **Mummylicious** doesn't mean that you spend hours in front of the mirror or at the gym while you neglect to care for your children at home. Your family and your children are your top priority, but you nurture them without losing your sense of self, or giving up on your figure and on your looks. Judy Garland summed it up best when she declared: "Always be a first-rate version of yourself, instead of a second-rate version of someone else."

Find your own unique style – your distinct brand of beauty and brains. It's about embracing motherhood and also taking care of yourself physically, mentally and emotionally. Being **Mummylicious** is being disciplined; it's knowing how to prioritize and be practical, without ever losing that sense of "coquetterie" (as the French describe it) – that desire to look pretty, seductive and feminine.

Lastly and most importantly, being **Mummylicious** means being a woman who loves and respects herself.

What the Hell Happened to My Body? Your Post-Delivery Body: Appraising the Situation and Measuring Up

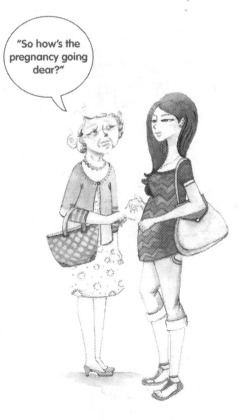

"So how's the pregnancy going dear?"

So now you're back home with your bundle of joy, and it's the most incredible feeling. You have succeeded in creating another human being, and you and your partner are both walking on air. Nine months of waiting at long last over, and you're cooing with pride and marveling at your baby's gorgeous little features.

Whether you've had an easy or difficult pregnancy, you are almost certainly relieved that it's finally over, with the last few weeks of gestation having been particularly tiresome and uncomfortable. You may even feel slimmer, compared to your body the weeks before delivery, now that you don't have that big bowling ball between your breasts and legs. I was especially proud of myself in the hospital shower when I realized I could touch my toes again without falling over.

That sense of euphoria quickly evaporated a week later, when in my apartment lift, a well-meaning neighbour accidentally asked me how the pregnancy was going. With dismay, I immediately understood that to others, I still looked four or five months pregnant. And even if this is normal - given that a post-pregnancy uterus remains quite distended the first few weeks after delivery - it made me cringe with embarrassment.

After you come down from your cloud of new-baby happiness long enough to take a good look at your post-delivery body and assess the damage, be prepared to take stock without being too harsh on yourself. Your body has been through a lot. Making a baby is no small task. You need to give your body time to heal and regroup. I often think of a pregnant woman's body as a piano accordion. It's incredible how our bodies can stretch and grow to an incredible volume and shape, and yet never lose its potential to shrink back to its original size.

Thus in your own good time, and when you feel ready, begin by taking an honest look at your post-delivery figure. Choose a moment when your little angel is fast asleep, and go and stand in front of a mirror. You might want to lock your door before you do this, in case you frighten anyone who might be wandering in. Now remove all your clothing and take a long hard look.

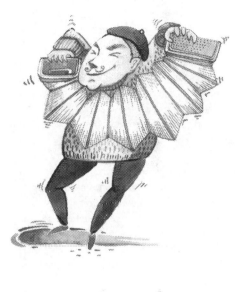

Your Feet and Legs

There is a very good chance that they may appear bloated and heavy. Your once-shapely ankles and feet could feel like they have almost doubled in size. It's very common for pregnant women to go up a shoe size, but most of the volume, if not all, can be attributed to water retention. The extra pressure caused by the weight gain and your strained circulation might have also given you small varicose veins, or spider veins as they are sometimes called, at the back of your legs. These may subside partially in time, as you shed the weight and excess water. If they do persist and still bother you, you could consider taking a trip to the phlebologist to make them disappear permanently.

Your Thighs and Buttocks

During all of my pregnancies, not once was my husband ever allowed to take a good look at my naked bottom. If he happened to catch a glimpse of it accidentally reflected in a mirror, it would send me into an embarrassed and fuming protest, which would in turn have him in fits of laughter – to my utmost dismay. From the first few weeks of pregnancy, I was convinced I was retaining water. And despite my best efforts, as the nausea set in and my intake of carbohydrates increased to placate my queasiness, the weight quickly started piling on. Thus, when climbing out of bed naked, I would walk out of the room backwards, at the risk of tripping over, so as to avoid a chance peek at my rapidly expanding, cellulite-dimpled bottom.

It didn't help that when I was a child, I had the misfortune of accidentally walking into our guest bathroom and catching sight of our sweet but very fat houseguest's naked behind, as she was brushing her teeth in the sink. Since I was the height of her bottom then as well, I never forgot this God-awful sight. It scarred me for life and gave me a phobia of cellulite, hence the rear-ward style of my exits from the conjugal chamber.

A post-pregnancy bottom - after nine months of pregnancy hormones, weight gain and water retention - well, let's just say it as it is, it is NOT a pretty sight. As ridiculous as it sounds, the first time I really looked at my bottom and thighs in the mirror after delivery, I cried. Cellulite was rampant, like bad cottage cheese gone wild and the once pert bottom I was so proud of was a shapeless mass of fat, resembling two bowls of upturned English jelly which no one wanted to eat.

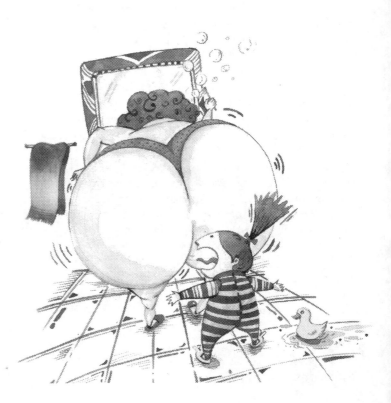

But let me quickly add that your thighs and bottom are where your body has stored the most fat during pregnancy, so as to create a reserve for the production of rich and precious breast milk for your baby's nourishment. This landmine of cellulite and fat has a higher purpose, which is to feed your treasured cherub. So let's just say that it may be best to leave it as is, for the moment.

Your Hips

Your hips may also appear unusually wide at this time, and that's completely natural and to be expected. During the third trimester, pregnancy hormones cause the ligaments holding the pelvic girdle together to soften, allowing the birth canal to widen during labour and delivery. As the pregnancy progresses and you gain additional weight, more fat collects on the outside of the hips. The good news is that the redistribution of "wealth" around your waist can be controlled through diet and exercise in the months to come, and the looser ligaments will firm up over time, but your pelvis may or may not return to its exact pre-pregnancy shape. This, of course, depends on a number of factors – on how wide or narrow your hips were before pregnancy, on how big your baby was at birth and on whether you've had a vaginal or C-section type delivery. But with determination and patience, there is a very good chance that your hips will revert to their original width or at least come very close to their previous size.

Your Belly

Despite its new shapelessness, your belly is not as big as it was before. So there is some good news here, after all. You might still look about four months pregnant because of your distended uterus. And your tummy may somehow feel like the Banaue rice terraces of the Philippines, with layers of fat and flab sitting loosely in folds around your abdomen, but as my Mum used to kindly point out, "At least, dearie, you no longer look like an anaconda that swallowed a small calf."

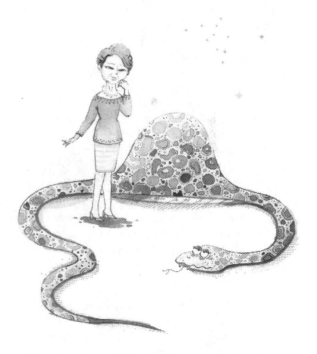

If you had a C-section, your belly will not only have these folds, but also an incision above your pubic area. And since you have absolutely zero muscle tone in that region after pregnancy, your folds will be at the complete mercy of gravity, shifting with you in the bed as you roll around trying to get comfortable.

During pregnancy, most women also develop a linea nigra, or a dark line in the centre of the tummy. Since it is hormone-induced, the longer you breastfeed, the longer it will take the linea nigra to disappear. It is the same pregnancy hormone (melanin) that causes the pigments of the skin on your nipples to darken, but these, too, revert to their original colour and size after about six to twelve months.

On average, 50% to 70% of women get stretch marks during pregnancy, and most of these will be on the tummy, although some women may also get a few on the thighs, breasts and hips. No one really knows why some women get them and others don't. Research suggests that genetics play a role. If your mother or sister got stretch marks during pregnancy, you're more likely to as well. No amount of cream or oil can prevent them. Of course, moisturizing your skin helps keep it more supple and less itchy during pregnancy. And trying to control how quickly you put on weight could also help, but at the end of the day, if you are meant to have them, they will appear. And as infuriating as it is, there is nothing you can do to prevent them.

Thus, when you inspect your post-delivery body and come to terms with the reality of stretch marks, if indeed you have developed some, be brave, my sister, and count these as battle scars on the way to motherhood. Your little angel is worth it all, and stretch marks won't prevent you from regaining your figure or strutting on the beach in a sexy maillot.

The good news is that stretch marks usually turn out to be considerably less noticeable six to twelve months after childbirth. The pigmentation fades, and they generally become lighter than the surrounding skin (the colour will vary depending on your skin tone), but their texture will remain the same. You won't be able to banish them altogether, but if your stretch marks still bother you after your pregnancy, talk to a dermatologist about ways to minimize them.

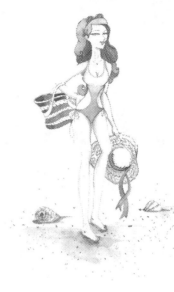

Your Breasts

One thing that cheered me up after delivery was the sudden feeling that I must have been a famous exotic dancer in my past life. As the "breast fairy" arrived in our home and my milk came gushing in, my already enhanced pregnancy breasts suddenly became quite spectacular apparitions indeed. Moreover, as I stood naked scrutinizing my body after delivery, with its thick wobbly thighs and rice-terrace-like belly, trying hard to ignore the looming bottom behind me, I stood up proudly and realized for the first time in my life, "So this is what it means to be a big-breasted goddess." Despite the extremely uncomfortable feeling caused by engorgement, at least the large breasts helped balance out the thicker waistline, bottom and legs. Thus I began to visualize them as big pumps sucking out all the excess water and fat stored in my body during pregnancy. I am convinced that breasts are the best ally a new mother has on the road to regaining her pre-pregnancy figure. It's nature's way of helping you convert a large part of your excess fat and water into a highly nutritional substance for your baby. But more on the topic of breasts and breastfeeding in the next few chapters.

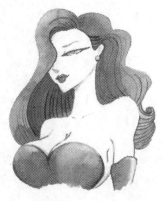

Your Face, Chin, Neck and Back

As much as my husband likes to disagree with me, post-delivery close-up pictures of us mothers should be banned. Those pictures should only feature the fruits of our labour (literally), our adorable little newborn baby. Part of the weight gain and water retention that come with pregnancy causes some women to develop very chubby cheeks and a generally rounder face. A number of us even get puffy eyes, not to mention red capillaries on the eyeballs and sometimes on the cheeks from the strain of pushing in the delivery room. In addition, fat seems to find its way and deposit itself on our face, chin and neck during the last trimester of pregnancy. Who knew that you could store fat on your neck and back?

I realized this for the first time in my life when, in my eighth month of pregnancy with my first child, I lifted my chin up and tilted my head back so as to pull my hair into a ponytail, when I discovered, to my horror, a small roll of fat at the base of my neck and upper back. Not only did I have to deal with being pregnant and generally heavier, but I also had chubby cheeks, an ominous double chin, a thicker neck and now, fat padding on my upper back. But let me reassure you once again that if you are, as I was, worried that the reflection in the mirror staring back at you strangely resembles a bloated and overweight chipmunk, that too undoubtedly will improve in time.

MEASURING UP

So now that you have completed the general inspection of your post-delivery body, with courage and honesty, reach for a measuring tape and standing as straight as you can, measure yourself:

Breasts - Yes, milk and all.

Waist - What waist? I hear you, but find the slimmest part you can.

Hips - At the thickest part, including your bottom.

Thighs - Also at the thickest part.

Write the date, your weight and your measurements on a little notebook or on the table provided at the end of this book, which you will keep and bring out every month to jot down your dimensions and progress as time goes by. And as depressing and futile as this exercise may appear to be today, it will only serve to show you how much progress you will have made and how far you will have come in terms of your figure in the next six to twelve months. Just look at it this way – you have to start somewhere, and at this stage, things can only get better. I've been there four times and done this every time. So read on and I'll tell you just how I got through it.

CHAPTER TWO

"THERE ARE THREE REASONS FOR BREASTFEEDING: THE MILK IS ALWAYS AT THE RIGHT TEMPERATURE; IT COMES IN ATTRACTIVE CONTAINERS; AND THE CAT CAN'T GET IT."

IRENA CHALMERS

Kick Starting Your Weight-Loss Program: What Breastfeeding Can and Can't Do for Your Figure

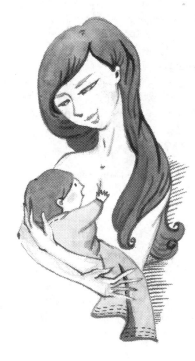

At the risk of sounding like a La Leche League supporter, I will only say this once: "Breast is best." Let me rephrase this – what I mean is that in addition to the proven benefits that breastfeeding can offer your newborn baby, it is also the best thing you can do for your figure immediately after giving birth. If you are lucky enough to be able to breastfeed and are willing to do it, then nature has provided us mothers with a way to not only feed our babies, but also regain the semblance of a figure immediately after birth.

Once you have adjusted and have gone beyond the discomfort of engorgement and eventually settled into the routine of nourishing your new baby, let nature take over. As your baby suckles on your nipples, it will cause your uterus to contract and help it shrink back to its original size. Nipple stimulation triggers the mother's brain to release the hormone oxytocin into the bloodstream. This hormone causes the muscles inside the vagina to contract, and this means that you will be one small step closer to getting a flatter tummy.

During the first few weeks of breastfeeding, a large part of the excess water which you were retaining will slowly be funneled to these magical pumps. In addition, breastfeeding burns around 500 to 600 calories a day. These abundant fat and water reserves which your body has accumulated over the past nine months will now come into play.

At this stage, you should be able to eat almost anything you want and not put on any weight at all. In fact, the first few weeks after delivery, you may even feel a surge of hunger as your stomach finds itself suddenly less compressed. That's ok. You will need energy to produce milk and get through the sleepless nights. Moreover, if you are breastfeeding, you will notice that in the first two to three weeks after delivery, you will most likely be losing about one pound (or about half a kilo) a week on average. But keep in mind that the weight loss immediately after birth is usually fluid loss. Thus don't forget to drink as much water as you can since breast milk is composed mostly of water. The current recommendation for breastfeeding mothers is to drink at least eight glasses of water a day.

The first few days after giving birth, your breasts will produce more colostrum – the same thick yellowish fluid which leaked from your breasts while you were pregnant that is rich in protein and antibodies. This precious substance, also called baby caviar, is truly worth its weight in gold. Not only is it rich-tasting and highly nutritional, but feeding your baby this substance will also help his digestive system get ready for breast milk, and give him passive immunity for the first few months of life. Over time, the milk will evolve from thin, watery and sweet, to thick, creamy and high in carbohydrates.

Breastfeeding your baby is a fantastic calorie-burner which allows you to eat what you want and still lose weight. You shouldn't go on a diet at this stage or even exercise vigorously because this may cause your body to release higher levels of toxins into your breast milk. For mothers who decide to breastfeed for longer periods of time, for over a year to 18 months for instance, dieting and vigorous exercise is not advisable. Remember that the nutrients your baby needs will be pulled from your body into your breast milk no matter what. If you aren't replacing those nutrients from your diet, you'll find your own reserves depleted too fast. And that could almost assuredly affect your health, energy level and your baby's milk supply. Nursing is a privileged moment for both mother and baby, which you should both enjoy and take pleasure in. So sit back, relax and enjoy the ride - let nature work its magic!

What you CAN do at this stage, to slowly and safely start your weight-loss program are the following two things:

1. Eat smart

2. Increase your activity level

Eat Smart

Even though you should be able to eat almost anything and not gain any weight, breastfeeding is NOT a license to binge and stuff your face. It doesn't give you a permit to devour all your favourite foods on any occasion. You should eat healthily and as normally as possible. "Eat to hunger" is the recommended guideline, or eat when you are hungry and until you feel satisfied. Stay away from too many deserts, junk food or fried foods. Opt for fresher and healthier alternatives. The ideal solution at this stage is to continue to eat a healthy balanced diet, with an abundance of vegetables and fruit; full-grain cereals, breads and pastas; and lean meat and fish. Eating this way while breastfeeding will put your body on the right track to a gradual healthy weight loss.

Even moderate restraint with your diet during lactation can help you lose about four or five pounds a month. Mothers who breastfeed more frequently lose weight faster than those who nurse less often. And mothers who nurse for shorter periods of time tend to lose weight more slowly than mothers who nurse longer. But you may get lucky and still find that you can eat more than you ever could before, and still lose weight while nursing.

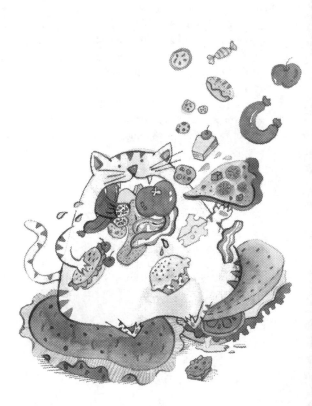

Increase Your Activity Level

Moderate exercise is extremely beneficial for nursing mothers. But it is essential to check with your doctor first before beginning any kind of postpartum exercise, especially if you've had a C-section or a difficult birth. If you've had a normal vaginal birth and have received the green light from your practitioner, there should be no impediment to beginning a light exercise program three to six weeks after delivery.

The only exercise I recommend at this early stage, which you can begin a few weeks after delivery, is walking. I used to think that walking, like golf, was an "old" person's activity. Walking for me was just something I did when I wanted to get from point A to point B. But when I realized that I wanted to start getting fit while still breastfeeding my babies and moreover, when I understood that running up to the tennis net for an overhead smash with breasts full of milk could get me knocked out rather than get me the point, walking quickly began to look like the best fitness option after all.

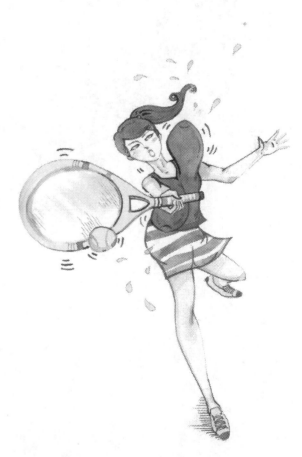

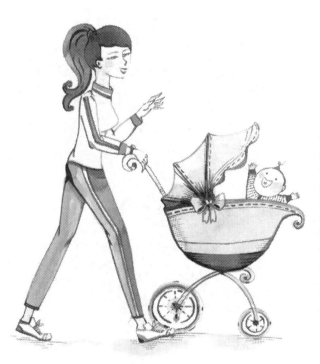

Walking is not only an excellent exercise for maintaining health, but also one of the best activities to help control weight. Permanent fat loss will take time. Even though calories do matter, it's not just about burning as many calories as possible, especially during the beginning stages of weight loss. To lose weight, it is vital to start off with an exercise that will help burn fat directly, one which also helps to slowly develop fitness levels so that higher-calorie-burning exercises may be performed later on in the program, in order to speed up weight loss.

Walking is probably the best exercise to start losing permanent weight for post-delivery mothers. It will help tone your legs and bottom, it will increase your fitness by raising your heart rate moderately and it should cause you to sweat, which releases toxins, clears the pores and helps you process some of your excess water weight. Plan to exercise after nursing so your breasts won't be full and uncomfortable. Wear a supportive sports bra and a pair of good walking shoes. Be sure to do some basic stretches to reduce muscle tension before you go on your regular walks. Drink a glass of water before and immediately after exercising. And drink more in hot weather.

Take walks with your baby in his or her pram or in a baby carrier. The baby's extra weight will use up even more calories. If there are other new mums in your neighbourhood, you can organize a group to go for regular morning walks together. This will help keep you motivated and make the outings more enjoyable. Walking, whether with a group or on your own, is easier to fit into your daily schedule as it allows you to take your baby with you. Weather permitting, go for a walk every day. This counts as exercise and gets you out of the house as well. If the weather keeps you inside and you don't have access to a treadmill, try carrying your little one in a sling while you walk around the house doing chores. You may feel silly, but the baby will love it anyway.

If you have access to a treadmill and if someone can watch your baby for 30 or 40 minutes, I recommend a brisk walk at a medium incline (level three or four) every day. It should feel as if you are walking up a very small hill. Three weeks after delivery, I started walking on a treadmill every morning for about 30 minutes at a medium incline and at a comfortable speed. Then over a period of several weeks, I gradually worked my way up to the maximum incline (15) and at a slightly faster pace. I could feel my body slowly toning up and my muscles coming alive. Sweating felt wonderful, too, and the exercise was very relaxing. In addition, this short time away from the baby was a healthy break and a precious moment to focus on myself and on my body. Moderate exercise such as this during your breastfeeding months will not only be good for your general fitness, but will give you more energy to deal with the sleepless nights and the overall mental and physical fatigue of the first few months after the birth. Once you finally stop breastfeeding, you can then begin a more vigorous exercise program and start dieting.

I breastfed each of my four children for about three to four months. But every mother must decide what works best for her and her baby. Deciding to breastfeed is a very personal choice, and how long you want to do it for must not be decided by anyone but yourself. You mustn't be pressured either way. Breastfeeding has been proven to have numerous benefits for both mother and baby, but it may not be everyone's cup of tea. It does help you lose some of the weight you gained during pregnancy, but breastfeeding in itself is NOT a weight-loss program. If you want to lose the weight, breastfeeding may help at the onset, but only to a certain extent. You'll notice that after the initial steady weight loss of the first few months, this gradually slows down. Your body cannot rid itself of all of its fat reserves while you are breastfeeding. The hormones in your system necessary to maintain breastfeeding will force your body to retain some weight in order to sustain a healthy production of milk. Very often, it is only when breastfeeding stops completely and your menstrual cycle begins anew that the weight starts to really come off. That is why it is not advisable to go on a diet and exercise vigorously in order to lose weight while you are still breastfeeding. But before we continue, I want to share a little more on breasts and breast care while breastfeeding.

CHAPTER THREE

"I WAS THE FIRST WOMAN TO BURN HER BRA, BUT IT TOOK THE FIRE DEPARTMENT FOUR DAYS TO PUT IT OUT."

DOLLY PARTON

Weapons of Mass Lactation: Your Breasts and Damage Control While Breastfeeding

In all likelihood, your breasts will have gone up a full cup since you got pregnant. And let's face it, for a lot of women, one of the advantages of being pregnant is the enhanced cleavage. Most husbands will tell you that they love you regardless, but that more cleavage and bigger breasts are a nice pregnancy bonus. That said, after delivery and as the milk engorgement takes over those already sizeable globes, your pride in their newly increased size may quickly turn to resentment and even disbelief. In fact, having engorged, rock-hard and painful breasts with leaking nipples, which cause you to smell like croissants and warm sour milk, is probably the least sexy feeling in the world. I know it made me want to kick someone in frustration every time it happened, no matter how mentally prepared I was for it. Engorgement usually takes place when colostrum changes to milk. However, it may also happen later if lactating mothers miss or skip several nursings, and not enough milk is expressed from the breasts. This can bring about swelling, throbbing and may even cause extreme pain. So when engorgement actually takes place, not only might you feel like your breasts are no longer your own, but the excruciating agony, discomfort and leakage associated with it may also make you wish you had never agreed to embark on this baby-feeding scheme in the first place.

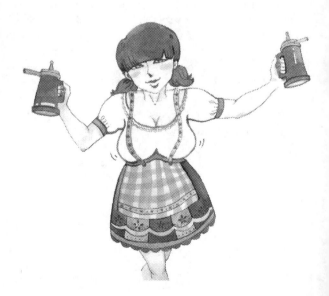

Hold Up Your Assets

At this point, I cannot convey strongly enough how important it is to be wearing a supportive bra. The skin on the breasts is incredibly delicate and too much engorgement and strain may cause stretch marks to appear. You may use a regular bra, which you can take off when you breastfeed, or a nursing bra with breast flaps. Cotton bras are best as they will not trap moisture that can irritate your nipples. Avoid wearing underwire bras. Your milk ducts extend up towards your armpits and underwire bras can squeeze your breasts and pinch milk ducts, causing plugged ducts or mastitis (breast infection). Make sure your bra fits correctly and does not squeeze your breasts. I found that regular sports bras gave me the most comfortable and best support. Thus I slept with one and never took it off, except to shower, throughout all my months of breastfeeding. This is also the time when you will need a breast pump to help alleviate engorgement, since a newborn baby's hunger may not always be enough to relieve the pressure.

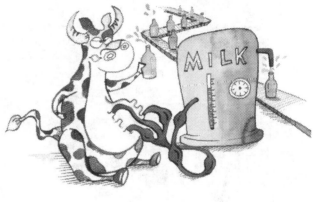

The Breast Pump

Enter stage right: The Breast Pump. Here's another torture device, which although designed to assist us women, brings us the closest yet to feeling like a cow being milked. One of the things that in my opinion can really turn a man off breasts (yours, in this case) – and let's face it, not many things can – it is the sight of his wife's breasts stuffed into the nozzle of one of these contraptions. Breast pumps literally vacuum your nipples until they feel like they are being ripped off your body, just so that you may extract a few milliliters of precious breast milk. And as if nine months of pregnancy, giving birth and breast engorgement weren't already giving enough discomfort, many women unfortunately need to add plugged milk ducts and sore cracked nipples to the list of risks associated with the running of the "all-night milk bar."

Plugged Milk Ducts

If you're making milk faster than it's getting expressed, it can get backed up in one of the ducts. When this happens, the tissue around the duct becomes swollen and inflamed, causing a blockage. The first sign of a plugged duct may be a small, hard lump that's sore to the touch or a very tender spot in your breast. Some women also notice redness in a particular area on their breast. The spot may feel hot or swollen, but will feel better after nursing. The best thing to do in this case is to place a warm, moist facecloth on the area for two to five minutes. Gently massage behind the plugged duct towards the nipple area while breastfeeding. This will help the flow of milk. If breast swelling, redness, increased pain or a fever develops, please seek medical attention immediately.

Nipple Care

It is normal to experience slight nipple tenderness when baby latches on in the first three to five days after birth. After that, proper positioning and latch-on techniques should help prevent nipple soreness. Many mothers experience rapid relief from nipple pain when they begin to position the baby properly. Most ointments sold for nipple soreness are not particularly useful in my opinion, and some may even be harmful to the baby's digestive system, so avoid them if possible. Certain women find that putting a little breast milk on the nipples after each feed helps protect the nipples and alleviate the pain.

Weaning Your Baby – The Key to Letting Your Breasts Adjust

Ideally, weaning should be a gradual process and should take a few weeks to a couple of months. Abrupt weaning, unless it is for urgent medical reasons, should always be avoided for the sake of both you and your baby. Unexpectedly taking away the breast can be very disturbing for the baby, since nursing is not only a food supply for him or her, but also a source of security and emotional comfort. The longer you give your breasts time to adjust to the weaning process, the better they will recalibrate and emerge from this transition in the best shape possible, so to speak.

My recommendation is to eliminate a feed and to give your body at least a week or two to adjust each time. Subsequently, continue by getting rid of another feed and letting a couple more weeks elapse. Go along with this process in a slow and gradual manner, giving your baby and your breasts time to adjust every time, until you are no longer breastfeeding and have replaced all feeds with the bottle.

You may notice some sagging in your breasts immediately after you have completely terminated the weaning process, and some women say this is inevitable. But it also largely depends on your skin type, how big your pre-pregnancy breasts were, how long you breastfed your baby and what kind of support you gave your breasts throughout your pregnancy and breastfeeding months. In fact, each woman may have a very different experience in terms of what happens to her breasts after breastfeeding. Some very lucky ladies don't even notice much of a change at all, and this is usually the case with women who start out with more modest or smaller-sized breasts.

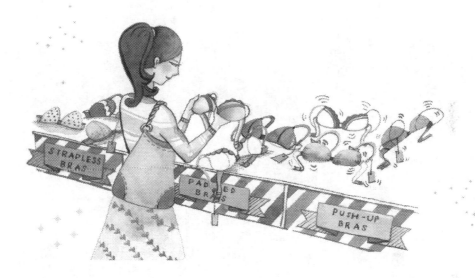

While on the contrary, other women's breasts never really recover and end up sagging dramatically - sometimes also comically referred to as "chesticles," as in saggy breasts that resemble testicles. The good news is that most women simply end up with slightly smaller and somewhat less firm breasts. What tends to happen is that the tissue inside the breasts shrinks after the weaning process, while the skin surrounding it doesn't, thus the breasts can sometimes appear a little deflated. After the weaning process, a woman's body does usually deposit some fat back into the breasts (this process typically takes many months), so that they may regain part of their pre-pregnancy size, but unfortunately some slight sagging usually remains.

Once you have totally weaned your baby, give the skin on your breasts time to get used to their new weight and size. In general, it takes skin many months to adjust to a new body shape, and although the forces of gravity cannot totally be reversed, certain chest exercises which work the muscles around the breasts can strengthen and help give them a firmer and more defined appearance. Of course, push-up bras can also do wonders to give your breasts that added visual pertness, and there are many creams on the market that claim to help firm up breast tissue. But short of running to a plastic surgeon, know that improving your posture can delay the impression of sagging. This involves working the core muscles or taking postural alignment classes such as Pilates.

CHAPTER FOUR

"THERE ARE NO SHORTCUTS TO ANY PLACE WORTH GOING."

BEVERLY SILLS

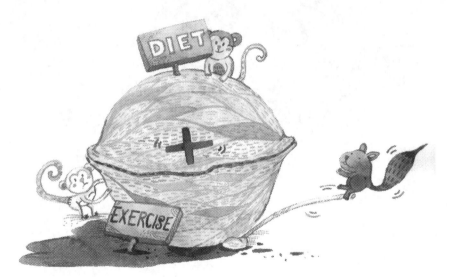

The Mummylicous Weight-Loss Combo – in a Nutshell

Now that you have successfully managed to wean your baby off breast milk and your body has adjusted to your post-breastfeeding self, you most probably have a certain amount of weight which you still want to lose. Be it five, 10, 15 kilos or more, in my experience this weight is the most challenging to shed.

Nevertheless, the key behind the **Mummylicious** Weight-Loss Program is very straightforward. To put it in the simplest terms - and we are not reinventing the wheel here - **it is to burn more calories than you consume every day**. When this takes place, your body will tap into those remaining stubborn fat reserves and convert them into fuel, which in turn will result in a gradually slimmer and happier you. For all intents and purposes, that's what it boils down to. How you go about getting this result is, of course, another matter altogether.

Two Crucial Elements: Diet and Exercise

For your body to burn more calories than you consume every day over a period of many months, it is essential that you combine the two key elements which will trigger and maintain your gradual weight reduction at a steady pace: diet and exercise. In the long term, one without the other makes each almost futile, in my view. But both combined and calibrated to perfection results in a formidable figure-shaping team which can do phenomenal things for your body. The bottom line concerning calories and weight loss is very simple. If we burn more calories than we consume, we will lose weight. If we consume more calories than we burn, we will gain weight. There are no shortcuts. The trick is to find the balance using both diet and exercise.

Dieting without any exercise at all results in you losing muscle tissue first, before fat, and consequently you end up with a lower metabolism and a somewhat weaker and flabbier body. Even if you may appear to be losing weight on the scales, it is not a good long-term solution and can be detrimental to your overall health and figure.

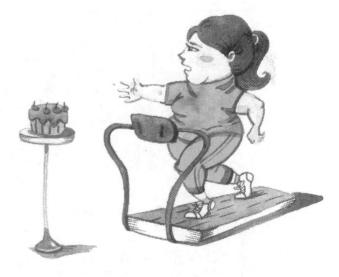

On the other hand, exercising without a sensible diet plan may result in you losing no weight at all and actually putting on some weight, which can be incredibly depressing, even if some of it may be attributed to muscle weight. So the key is to embark on this weight-loss journey convinced that you need both of these elements to succeed. But being merely convinced won't be sufficient. Before you move forward with this program, as with any major project, you will need to be crystal-clear about your goals and objectives – and, more importantly, 100% convinced and decided in terms of your commitment level.

CHAPTER FIVE

"IN EVERYTHING, THE ENDS WELL DEFINED ARE THE SECRET OF DURABLE SUCCESS."

VICTOR COUSINS

The Mummylicious Acid Test:
Fitting Into Those Old Jeans Again Setting an Achievable Weight Goal And Timeline

For some strange reason, six weeks after giving birth to my second child, I had the crazy idea to try on my favourite pair of jeans. I must have been feeling particularly delusional that day because I proceeded to stuff my legs into them. I managed to get the jeans halfway up above my knees, and as I was hopping around desperately trying to pull them on, I fell over forward and nearly knocked myself unconscious against the dressing room cupboard. What was I thinking? This obviously premature attempt crystallized in my mind what my real objective was.

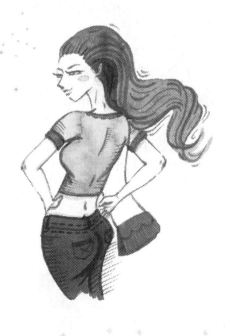

Jeans and a woman's figure - well, it's the ultimate acid test. How good a woman looks in her jeans is indicative of the real state of her figure. You can't hide much when you're wearing jeans. So use your favourite pair of jeans as a tool to help you decide what your target dream weight should be.

By the time we become adults, most of us women know deep inside what the best weight for our height should be. We know what that magical number is. It is the weight we were when we felt at our happiest and most satisfied with our figures. And regardless of what it is, it needs to be a number you will be comfortable aiming for today.

Don't focus on your BMI (Body Mass Index – body weight divided by the square of your height). There are many websites that can help you calculate it. In my view, the BMI should only be used as a general guideline. Keep in mind that it doesn't take into account your percentage of body fat versus muscle tissue and more importantly, it also doesn't allow for the fact that we all have different body frames, bone dimensions and density. Your ideal weight needs to be what will make YOU happy. Not what you think your friends, society, magazines and billboards advocate or even what your BMI says it should be.

This part is extremely important. Before you begin this weight-loss program, be true to yourself and very honest in terms of your goal, but do not be afraid to set the bar high. Some friends might tell you that your ideal weight is too low or too high. Everyone will have an opinion on your weight-loss objective, but ultimately it's not about what they think is right for you. Only YOU can decide that for yourself. So filter all those views out and stay focused on your own objective. Remember to set your goal high and commit to not stopping until you get there. Now write down you ideal weight in a place you will consult regularly. Be it your agenda, your calendar, your bathroom mirror or in the **Mummylicious** Weight-Loss Contract provided at the back of this book. This number should be as good as tattooed on the inside of your head. I used to find ways to be reminded of my ideal weight everyday by making it my password on my computer. This is exactly the kind of obsessive focus you need to succeed in your weight-loss endeavor.

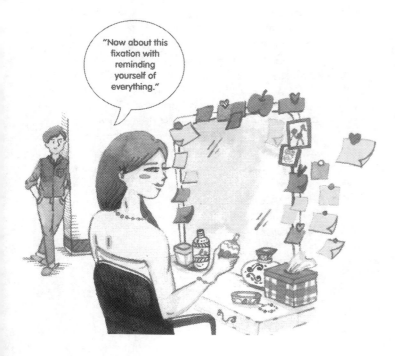

Your Timeline

Now for the timeline. They say the rule of thumb with pregnancy weight is nine months to put it on and nine months to take it off. This is too simplistic. Many factors can affect the time it will take you to get to your ideal weight – from how much weight you've put on during pregnancy to what your actual weight goal is, or how long you've decide to breastfeed to how much time you have to devote to weekly exercise, for example. When setting a timeline for yourself, it is important to have a goal that is realistic and attainable. It may take some people six months, 18 months, two years or even more to get back to their ideal weight. The important part is not how fast you get there, but actually just getting there and maintaining it at that level.

In short, you must stay committed to your decision but stay flexible with your timeline. A year might seem long in your mind, but the first year of having a baby, as most mothers will tell you, will fly by so fast, you won't even know what hit you. Visualizing yourself at your baby's first birthday party, or attending a friend's wedding, for example, looking slimmer and happy, could just be the incentive to get you started.

From the time I stopped breastfeeding my children to the time I reached my ideal weight goal, it has generally taken me between six to 12 months. This is committing to, on average, at least four exercise sessions a week and sticking to the **Mummylicious** Diet Plan. My advice is to give yourself at least nine to 12 months minimum, and more, if you have a sizeable amount of weight to drop. Remember, getting there eventually, is what matters – not the time it takes you. If you have given yourself 10 months to lose 10 kilos (22 pounds), for instance, you need to cut the time into little segments. Depending on how fast or slow you see the weight start to come off, you can recalibrate accordingly. So by the halfway mark, at the fifth month, you will need to have lost five kilos (11 pounds). This means that, on average, you must lose one kilo (2.2 pounds) a month. And remember that your timeline is not rigid. It can be slightly lengthened or shortened, depending on your needs and weight-loss rate.

That said, losing weight too fast is not advisable. If you try to pressure your body into dropping the pounds faster than it naturally wants to, you can cause significant damage to your health. Rapid weight loss leads to fatigue and drains your energy levels and stamina. Losing weight quickly takes its toll on your appearance, causing your skin to dry out, your hair to lose its luster and your complexion to appear gaunt. Although most dieters are in a hurry to lose weight, a slow but gradual weight loss is always the best for two simple reasons. Slower weight loss lasts longer, and it teaches dieters good eating habits. Rather than considering your weight-loss program as just a diet, think of it as a lifetime weight-control eating system. Too many dieters determine to lose weight by a certain date and then slowly put the weight back on as they go back to their old eating habits. Rather than adopting this mind-set, simply decide to change eating habits for a lifetime, instead of a small chunk of time. And although it can be very motivational to have a particular date or event in mind, it's really not about a quick fix, but more about focusing on developing healthier long-term eating patterns.

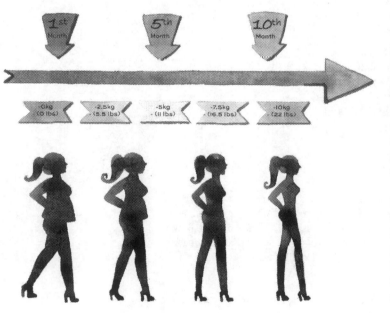

When you set out to lose weight slowly, there may not be instantly noticeable changes on the scale day after day. You are making sacrifices and getting only small rewards in return. This may be frustrating and leads you to wonder if the changes are really worth the effort. But focus on the bigger picture and imagine yourself looking svelte and fit at your child's 18-month checkup, for instance. These sacrifices gain more meaning, and the time it took for you to get fit becomes almost irrelevant. It's the lasting result that really matters.

Once you have decided on your ideal weight-loss number and designed a workable timeline, it is important to sketch a rough picture to help you visualize your step-by-step objectives. You need to see where you will be heading over the next few months, otherwise, a goal without a plan is simply a wish.

CHAPTER SIX

"IF I HAVE THE BELIEF THAT I CAN DO IT, I SHALL SURELY ACQUIRE THE CAPACITY TO DO IT."

GANDHI

The Importance of Strengthening Your Resolve and Willpower Visualizing Your Success + Making a Contract with Yourself

This is probably the most crucial chapter of the book. Embarking on a weight-loss program will have no meaning if you don't have the willpower and resolve to follow through with it. Ask yourself, "Do I really want to do this?" If the answer is a resounding yes, then the next two questions should be, "Am I willing to do what it takes to get to that dream weight?" and "Can I find the willpower to stick to this weight-loss program for as long as I need to, without making excuses and finding reasons to quit?"

You would be surprised at the number of people who say they wish they could lose weight but when push comes to shove are not willing to put up with the sacrifices needed to be successful in their endeavor. I won't deny that the next few months won't be a walk in the park, but the good news is that once you do reach your ideal weight, maintaining it won't be as hard. You won't have to be as strict with yourself, and my diet plan and exercise routine will help you maintain your figure for a lifetime, while still enjoying the good things in life.

Once you have decided that you are fully committed and moving forward with your weight-loss goals, you must reach deep inside yourself and strengthen your resolve. You need to believe that you can attain your goal and be willing to do what it takes. Sir Winston Churchill once declared, "It is no use saying, 'We are doing our best.' You have got to succeed in doing what is necessary." And as this great statesman once believed, it is about finding the real desire and means to accomplish your goal. You must believe that the results will make you proud and that the sacrifices along the way pale in comparison to the pleasure you will feel once you attain your objective.

It is interesting to reflect for a moment on what the word "resolve" actually means. Resolve is a steering mechanism that keeps us committed to staying on course. It makes us do things, accomplish goals and achieve objectives, and it is resolve that puts us into action. Robert Silverstone, a renowned seminar leader and professional coach, once declared that without it, "we'd be like a ship without a rudder, drifting aimlessly on the ocean of life, and the real power of resolve is located much deeper than the mind. It resides in the intuition, in the heart, in the spirit and in every cell of our being. We don't think about resolve … we feel resolve ... we are resolved!" So the true power of resolve is found in the present moment. What diminishes or weakens our resolve? Victim behaviour - such as blaming, thinking negatively, complaining and making constant excuses, finding reasons why we can't succeed - will only serve to weaken or diminish our resolve. What strengthens our resolve?

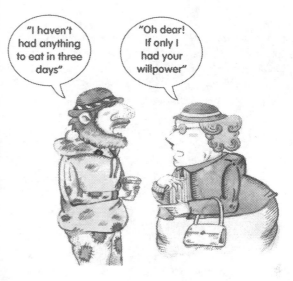

When we are confident and feel good about ourselves, when we have the courage of our convictions, when we are free of doubts and when we know that our actions are steering us towards a greater goal.

Motivational speaker Anthony Robbins once proclaimed: "I believe life is constantly testing us for our level of commitment, and life's greatest rewards are reserved for those who demonstrate a never-ending commitment to act until they achieve. This level of resolve can move mountains, but it must be constant and consistent. As simplistic as this may sound, it is still the common denominator separating those who live their dreams from those who live in regret." Once again, before you embark on this weight-loss program, the most crucial piece of the puzzle is to truly question the strength of your resolve and your will to succeed. Because nothing less than unwavering focus and determination are what it will take to get there.

Visualizing Your Success

"Picture yourself vividly as winning and that alone will contribute immeasurably to success. Great living starts with a picture, held in your imagination, of what you would like to do or be." - Harry Emerson Fosdick.

Some call it "following their dreams" while others may call it a "mental rehearsal." If you want to lose weight, picture yourself going through the effort of losing weight and eventually getting there: shedding the fat, sweating at the gym and feeling good, seeing the weighing scale hit that lower number, wearing that favourite cocktail dress again, seeing your best "frenemy" turn green with envy - anything that will motivate you!

Picture it all and every day. By mentally projecting where you want to be, you're giving yourself a mental roadmap to follow. When you visualize your future success, you start to believe in it and you start to believe in yourself. When you start to believe, you will literally ignite your willpower.

So what is visualization? It's like a mental rehearsal of what you want to have happen (try not to visualize what you don't want, or you could be setting yourself up for disaster!). The bestselling book "The Secret" by Rhonda Byrne describes how powerful visualization can change your life. Imagining your goals and dreams can lead to actually experiencing them, because your body and even the universe responds to your mind. When you visualize, you rehearse how a problem can be solved, how a new idea could be implemented or what a piece of art looks, reads or sounds like. You mentally practice achieving and living your goal, which leads to the real thing.

When you visualize your goals, neuromuscular templates are created. These templates are patterns of mind-body reflexes that prepare you for what you are going to do. When you visualize, your muscles experience electrical impulses that correspond to the physical event you are imagining.

Take the talented pianist Liu Chi Kung, for instance. He was imprisoned for seven years during the Cultural Revolution; when he was released from prison, some say he played better than before. How is that possible without practicing? He said, "I did practice, every day. I rehearsed every piece I ever played, note by note, in my mind." Visualization is not only used by surgeons and athletes, but also by those undergoing physical rehabilitation and by cancer patients. Visualizing your goal takes you into a whole new realm - which can be frightening and strange, but much safer in the confines of your mind. You can practice examining your success from new angles with all sorts of different scenarios. Visualization also allows you to see the big picture, from the perspective of your family, friends, colleagues. The more you picture it in your mind, the more likely it is to become reality. If you're facing an obstacle you don't understand or haven't ever experienced, your intuition can work its magic. Your intuition will bring forward inspiration that you hadn't previously considered.

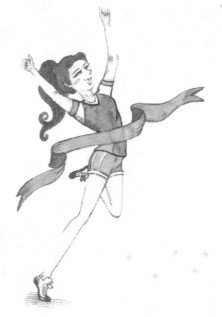

Making a Contract with Yourself

Here's the deal. You've decided on your ideal weight number. You have given yourself a timeline within which to get there, and you have thought long and hard about the strength of your resolve. Now comes the commitment part. You need to make a contract with yourself. Writing your goals down is a proven winning motivational tool to help you stick to your objective. When you do this, it is equally important to list the payoffs and benefits of reaching your goal. While losing weight is a benefit, you will want to list the reasons why you want to lose weight. Maybe the payoff is fitting into a certain dress again or looking great for an upcoming reunion. Perhaps it is because you want to improve your health or make your partner proud when he steps out with you to go to a party. Again, you should be specific when you set these benefits in your contract because it will help you stay motivated and will crystallize the visualization of your success.

List down the rewards. Rewards are important when you are setting goals for yourself. When you reflect on the rewards, think about the fun things that you will accomplish by reaching your goals. Lose that weight and look hot in your bathing suit or your favourite jeans. Whatever you think is the best part about reaching your goal, use that as a reward to help you stay motivated. The longer the list of benefits and rewards, the better for you, since you will be able to read and reread it anytime to help keep your resolve strong.

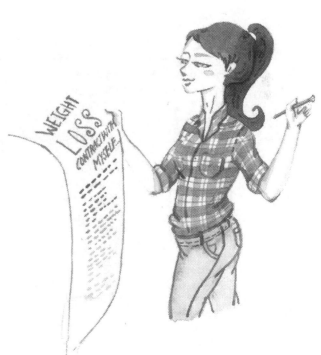

A key element of your contract is to have a specific action plan. An action plan will tell you what steps you need to take to reach your final goal. This part of the contract can be completed once you've finished reading this book (see the **Mummylicious** Weight-Loss Contract at the end of the book). List down what you need to change, do or accomplish in a day, a week, a month or a year. It will help keep you motivated to reach your end goal. Having a contract with a clear objective, timeline, a list of reasons why you are doing this and a list of rewards you plan to enjoy once you reach that goal, as well as a specific action plan which you will follow, will help you stay focused every day as you are moving towards your goal. How many times a week will you commit to exercising? How will you find a way to fit regular exercise into your schedule? What are certain foods and drinks that you will give up for a few months? Why are these sacrifices worth making? Remind yourself constantly why you are doing this for your body by writing it in your contract.

When you take the time to make an official contract with yourself, you will be motivated and ready to reach your goals. It will be easier when you can see your goals in writing and know what rewards and benefits are waiting for you along the way. Your action plan will help you to stay on track when you are working hard to accomplish your goals and dreams. Remember, it's character that got you started, commitment that moved you to action and discipline that will enable you to follow through and succeed.

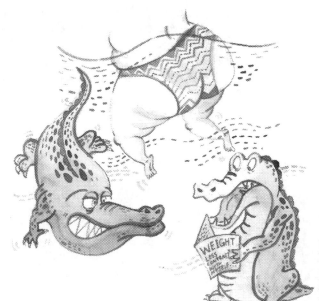

CHAPTER SEVEN

"NEVER EAT MORE THAN YOU CAN LIFT."

MISS PIGGY

The DIET:
Low Carbs and Portion-Control Combination

As described in Chapter Four, the main objective of the **Mummylicious** Weight-Loss Program is to burn more calories than you consume every day. This means you must consume less energy than what you expend through physical activity. One of the fastest ways to do this, of course, is to cut your calorie intake. And my recommended choice of diet is very simple. Essentially, it is a combination of low carbohydrates and portion control.

The low-carb diet (also called "reduced carbohydrate," "controlled carbohydrate" or "low glycemic" diet) is a broad term, encompassing many popular diets (such as Atkins, South Beach, Zone, Protein Power, Sugar Busters, Carbohydrate Addicts Diet) as well as eating plans that don't follow a rigid format but advise limiting the consumption of many foods that are high in carbohydrates.

The objective is NOT to cut all carbohydrates, since they provide important nutrition with vitamins, minerals and fibre which are essential for physical fitness and overall health, but only to limit the amount of WHITE carbohydrates, which include sugars and white starches (low in vitamins and minerals). A good guide is to try to eliminate, or greatly reduce, these five elements: white rice, potatoes, white pastas, white bread/cakes and sugar. Keep in mind that carbohydrates can also be found in many other foods: cereals, grains, fruit, beans, whole-wheat bread, oatmeal, some dairy products such as non-fat milk, plain yogurt, skimmed milk. So it would be almost impossible to remove them all and neither should you attempt to do this, since we need these kinds of "good" carbohydrates for our bodies to function in a healthy and efficient way. Additionally, it is interesting to learn more about what actually happens to our bodies when we lose body fat during a weight-loss program. What does it take for the body to reach into our fat reserves and use them as fuel, so that it results in actual weight loss? This state is called ketosis.

What Is Ketosis?

Ketosis is a stage in fat metabolism which occurs primarily when the body consumes little or no carbohydrates. When this happens, the body breaks down body fat for fuel, and this process results in three different molecules called "ketones" being released. Two of these molecules (acetoacetate and ß-hydroxybutyrate) can be used for fuel by most tissues of the body. The third molecule (acetone) cannot be broken down and used by the body, and thus it is excreted primarily in the urine. When you combine a low carbohydrate and portion-control eating plan with regular exercise as well as adequate lean protein, fruit, vegetables and a limited amount of carbohydrates, there is no need for the body to break down its own muscle tissue for fuel. Ketosis thus tends to accelerate fat loss without touching your muscle tissue. The key is to nourish yourself properly and to meet all your body's nutritional needs so that the body's muscles are spared and that only your body fat is broken down.

Ketosis allows the body to function efficiently and live off stored body fat when necessary. It makes the body run more economically and provides a backup fuel source for the brain. Being in ketosis by following a low carbohydrate diet is NOT dangerous. The human body was designed to use ketones very efficiently as fuel in the absence of glucose. However, the word ketosis is often confused with a similar word, ketoacidosis. Ketoacidosis is a dangerous condition for diabetics, and the main element is acid, not ketones. The blood pH becomes dangerously acidic because of an extremely high blood sugar level (the diabetic has no insulin, or doesn't produce enough insulin, so blood sugar rises, and it is the high blood sugar and the acid condition that is so dangerous). Ketosis is a metabolic state that occurs when your body has run out of carbohydrates and instead starts converting fat into ketones to use for energy. The key is to ensure that you are burning fat from your body stores, and that is why it is important that your protein intake be lean and low in fat, combined with lots of vegetables, grains, fibre and fruit.

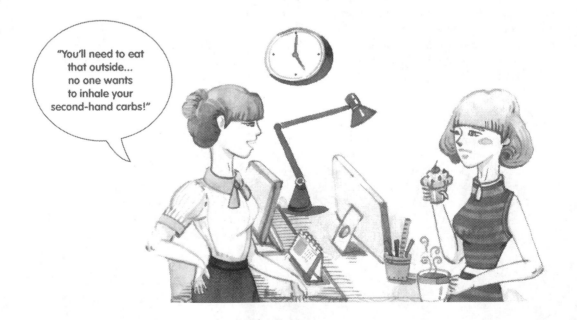

"You'll need to eat that outside... no one wants to inhale your second-hand carbs!"

In order to get rid of fat, other than by surgical means, we must force our body to break it down to use as a fuel source by consuming less energy or calories than what we expend through physical activity. In other words, body fat regulation is a matter of energy in versus energy out. That's about all you need to know to lose weight, though doing so in a healthy and gradual manner which can then be habit-forming is the key to success.

Being on a low-carb diet is not always easy. We all have our favourite starches that we enjoy. I myself am particularly fond of white rice, being half-Asian, and that is why I feel that the low-carb diet should sometimes be combined with a portion-control element, making it more sustainable for the long term. This means that if you find it hard to eliminate your main white starches completely – bread, rice, potatoes and pasta – then maybe a compromise can be reached.

Give yourself two or at the most three meals a week during which you are "allowed" to have your favourite white carbohydrate in moderation. This makes the diet much more worthwhile and easier to follow. A Friday night pasta or a Sunday morning pancake breakfast, for instance, were often my "rewards" for being "good" all week. Obviously, the key here is not to binge, but to eat these starches in reasonably small amounts.

My brother, who is a jujitsu athlete and a nutrition aficionado, once shared with me a recommended portion-control theory which he picked up during his research. He told me that when deciding on the size of your WHOLE meal portion, you mustn't eat more than what you can hold in the palm of your cupped hands. And when it comes to carbohydrates in particular, a SINGLE cupped hand portion is enough, or about the size of a tennis ball. And I've found that this is an excellent guideline when deciding on the amount of carbohydrates to consume on those days you allow yourself to have some. And at any rate, eating smaller portions on a daily basis long term is a good way to "train" your stomach to be satisfied with less. This will help you consume less calories as a result. Although technically the stomach doesn't actually shrink when you eat less, it does however adjust to smaller-portion meals over time.

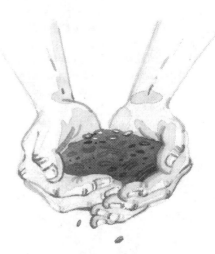

Does Caffeine Affect Ketosis?

There are a several studies that recommend avoiding caffeine because they say it may cause blood sugar to rise, with consequent effects on insulin, but many low-carbers continue to enjoy caffeine-containing beverages with no major impact on their weight-loss efforts. However, there are some sensitive individuals who are exceptionally insulin-resistant and consequently may need to limit or even remove all caffeine from their diet. If you have been losing weight successfully, then find that your weight loss has slowed down for a few months while following the program very accurately, you may consider discontinuing all caffeine for a while to see if that will get things under way once again.

Will Drinking Alcohol Affect Ketosis?

Yes and no. The liver can make ketones out of alcohol, so technically, when you drink, you'll keep on producing ketones and thus you will remain in ketosis. The problem is that alcohol transforms more easily to ketones than fatty acids, so your liver will use the alcohol first, in preference to fat. Thus, when you drink, basically your fat-burning state is suspended until all the alcohol is out of your system. This rapid breakdown of alcohol into ketones and acetaldehyde (the intoxicating by-product) seems to put low-carbers at risk of faster intoxication especially if no other food is consumed to slow down absorption.

To summarize, you must keep in mind that the simplest and most efficient way to cut your calorie intake without losing much nutritional benefits is to diminish your consumption of white carbohydrates. Additionally, you should try to consume lean protein such as fish, chicken, turkey and ham, combined with an abundance of vegetables and fruit. Some brown rice, whole-wheat bread and cereal, for instance, should be maintained in your diet, but in controlled quantities. Nevertheless, you will find that if you have too much of these complex carbohydrates, your weight-loss efforts could be neutralized or slowed down. So it may be best to consume them in small portions and earlier on during the day.

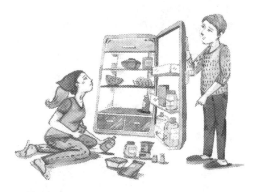

CHAPTER EIGHT

"LIVING A HEALTHY LIFESTYLE WILL ONLY DEPRIVE YOU OF POOR HEALTH, LETHARGY AND FAT."

JILL JOHNSON

The High-Fibre Breakfast

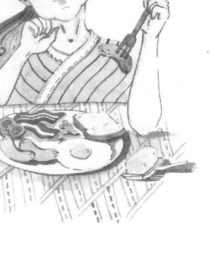

"Could it be my big breakfasts that are spoiling my diet? Or maybe I should also cut down on my big lunches, big dinners and big snacks..."

Many nutrition experts agree that breakfast is the most important meal of the day. Studies have shown that eating a healthy, nutritious breakfast everyday will lessen chronic disease and increase longevity. It boosts your energy, increases your attention span and heightens your sense of well-being, and provides at least one-third of your day's calories.

Our metabolism is designed to have a hearty breakfast and a lighter lunch and dinner. Additionally, it has been proven that if adults consume all of their daily calories in the morning, they lose weight, while if they consume the same amount at night, they gain weight. The enzymes in our body that help digest our food are at their peak levels in the mornings rather than later during the day. Our liver, which processes our food and therefore has a relationship with our energy level, likes to start slowing down in the late afternoon and early evening. By afternoon, the liver wants to start storing up energy for the next day (anabolic activity) rather than metabolizing food (catabolic activity). A small nutritional dinner, composed of some protein and vegetables, is much better tolerated than a dinner high in fats and loaded with carbohydrates (which often causes some people to get indigestion in the evenings). The key is to find a system that lets you have these types of breakfasts, lunches and dinners, but which also fits into your lifestyle as a family.

Breakfast is a great way to get more fibre into your diet, and a high-fibre diet doesn't only help reduce cholesterol, but also makes it easier for you to lose weight. The most fibre can be found in cereals with bran. Cereals such as Fibre One, All Bran and 100% Bran, for instance, are some of the highest in fibre. For those who prefer a better taste, Raisin Bran and Grape Nuts offer lower but adequate amounts of fibre. But the best way to compare products and find the best fibre is to read the product labels. Oatmeal is also very good for you and a favourite hot cereal for many. You can try a multi-grain cereal or granola as well and experiment with different grains such as millet, quinoa or corn grits for variety.

Choose fruit for breakfast, since fruit can also give you plenty of fibre. Fresh fruit is the best choice, and there are many to choose from: oranges, grapefruits, apples, bananas, grapes, kiwis, mangos, melons and berries. Canned fruit packed in juice is also a good choice as long as they are not too sweet. Add fresh or dried fruit and nuts to your cereal so as to make it more appetizing.

Breakfast has always been my favourite meal of the day. I take time and pleasure in eating my breakfast while reading the paper every morning. Often, I think of breakfast as an important pampering ritual for myself before the start of a busy day. So here are some breakfast ideas to help you kick start your day in the right and healthy way.

5 High-Fibre Breakfast Ideas

Raisin bran cereal (or other cereal) with low-fat milk and mixed berries

Hot oatmeal with low-fat milk, dried raisins and apples

Soft boiled egg and whole-wheat toast

Wild berry smoothie

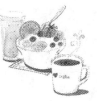

Stewed prunes with low-fat plain yogurt

All of the above can be accompanied with a glass of orange juice & a cup of tea or coffee (with low fat milk & no sugar)

CHAPTER NINE

"TO LENGTHEN YOUR LIFE, SHORTEN YOUR MEALS."

AUTHOR UNKNOWN

The Light Lunch

I sometimes think that lunch is the most challenging meal for a mother. It often seems to be the taken on the go. Whether you are working in an office (or from home) or are a stay-at-home mum, there never seems to be enough time to stop what you are doing during the day long enough to have a proper lunch. Yet lunch is a very important meal. Having a light lunch or snack can temporarily and greatly boost mental acuity. A large lunch, on the other hand, especially one very high in fat or carbohydrates, can increase the sluggishness that normally develops in the early afternoon.

Dieticians seem to agree that it is absolutely beneficial to take a lunch break. It's good for your mind as well as your spirit. Researchers believe that one of the reasons we sleep at night is that our brains need the downtime in order to rest and repair themselves. A lunch break gives your brains a similar opportunity. Emotionally, the lunch break provides you with time to get away from the cognitive demands of your job, your chores or other obligations, to relax a bit and recharge your emotional batteries.

The key is to eat the right foods so that you get the energy and nutrition without too many calories and fat. Being creative and selective with your lunches is the challenge at hand, but the right healthy light lunch will leave you feeling satisfied yet alert and full of energy for the rest of the afternoon. I have found that I prefer to eat a simple light lunch, which usually consists of a salad or a soup during the day while leaving the more complex dinner preparations for the evenings with the family.

My Mum used to say that we only have to look at our own teeth to understand what type of foods we as humans should really be consuming. "Most of our teeth are like those of a horse," she used to declare, "and we only have two canines" (which are there to help us cut through meat), so in her view, this clearly meant that we humans ought to eat a lot more "roughage," so to speak, rather than meat. I often think of her observation when I try to ensure I keep fruit and vegetables as top priorities and in abundant quantities in my daily diet plan.

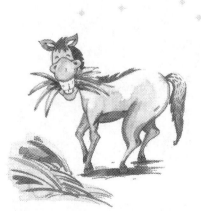

Light Lunch Ideas
6 Salads

Tuna Niçoise

Thai avocado, prawns and pomelo

Tomatoes, mozzarella cheese and fresh basil

Crispy Caesar with grilled chicken

Roasted pumpkin, baby spinach, pine nuts and ricotta cheese

Classic Greek

Pumpkin and apple

Broccoli and goat cheese

Wild mushroom with light crème

Chilled Gazpacho with creamy avocado

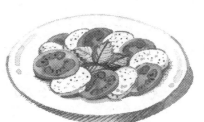

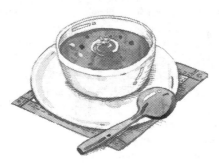

The wonderful thing about soups
is that you can always make a fresh batch
and keep it in the fridge,
or even freeze for future meals

"IF YOU CAN'T CONTROL YOUR PEANUT BUTTER, YOU CAN'T EXPECT TO CONTROL YOUR LIFE."

CALVIN AND HOBBES

The Dinner that Fits in with the Family

A household gets very busy when there are children around, and it seems that no other time of the day is as intense as bath time followed by dinner time. This moment is not called the "witching hour" by accident, with naked children running wild around the house, while the bathwater runs noisily. As you greet your partner when he walks in through the front door, you are trying to remember what you had planned to feed the family for dinner while, you hope, not looking too stressed and irritated with the children.

This is the reason why your **Mummylicious** Diet Dinner needs to fit around what you have planned for your family. It's very simple: whatever you've decide to cook for your family is what YOU will be having, too. The only difference is that your meal will be the "diet" version of theirs. And let's face it, it's not fun just having a salad while everyone else at the table is chomping on a delicious chili con carne. The key is to offer something delicious for your family but that can also be turned into a light diet dinner for you.

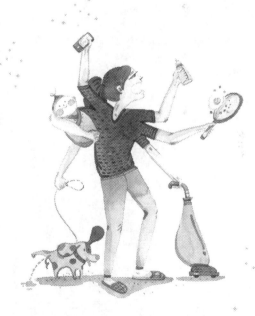

People usually give up on their diets because it is too hard to maintain and it doesn't fit into their daily lifestyle. For the diet to work for the long term, it needs to be sustainable and practical. If you prepare a delicious roast chicken for your family, for instance, have some by all means, but try not to touch the mashed potatoes (OK, have a tablespoon for the taste if you want), but be sure to have a generous serving of French beans or broccoli or whatever side vegetables you have prepared that night. This is the principle that you can apply every night at dinner time as you try to shed the excess weight over the next few months. Once you reach your target weight, you can begin to eat like the rest of the family again but always with a watchful eye on the amount of carbohydrates you consume.

10 Nutritional Dinner Ideas for You and the Family

Honey mustard glazed salmon fillets
and steamed French beans

Apricot chicken with fresh thyme
and steamed Brussels sprouts

Beef Bourguignon with pearl onions and
mushrooms, served with steamed carrots

Oven-cooked sea bass stuffed with fennel
and lemon, served with roasted olives
and tomatoes

Seafood bake served with
a crispy green salad

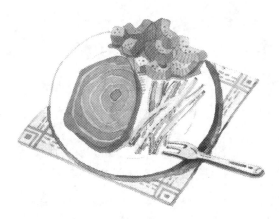

Chicken satay with peanut sauce
and roasted red peppers

Prawns cooked in coconut milk
and lime juice, served with steamed
green asparagus

Chicken croquettes with a cauliflower gratin

Stuffed bell peppers with ground beef,
corn and zucchini,
served with a crispy green salad

Roasted leg of lamb served with
flageolet beans and roasted tomatoes

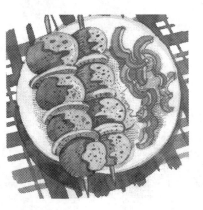

Of course for the rest of the family, you can serve these accompanied with rice, potatoes, couscous, pasta and any other kind of starches they like to eat. The tricky part for you will be to try to stay away from the carbohydrates as much as possible and simply have the fish, meat or poultry with a generous serving of vegetables or even a side salad of your choice (fresh tomatoes, or cucumbers in vinaigrette, for example). It will be hard the first few days and weeks, but after some time, your body will adjust to this kind of dinner. You will see that you won't miss the starches as much anymore, and dieting this way will become easier and easier as you see your weight come off on the scales.

The wonderful thing about this way of dieting is that you will be eating like the rest of the family with just a slight adjustment to your meal. Be sure to drink a lot of water during your meal so as to feel full sooner and not be tempted to attack the rice or mashed potatoes. This part will really test your willpower, but try to remember how happy you will feel when you start losing weight or when you finally fit into your favourite pair of jeans.

For the dishes listed in the previous pages, you can find recipes at the back of this book and also a few on my website (www.thesmartgirlshandbook.com).

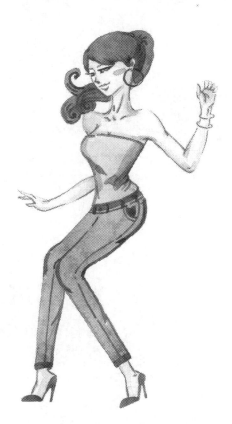

CHAPTER ELEVEN

"STRESSED SPELLED BACKWARDS IS DESSERTS. COINCIDENCE? I THINK NOT!"

AUTHOR UNKNOWN

Healthy Snacks + Drinks and Foods to Avoid

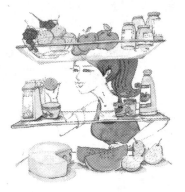

For women who are dieting, snacks often get eliminated in the name of saving calories. But snacking when you're watching your weight is actually a good idea as long as they are healthy snacks and in small controlled quantities. When dieting, people often wait too long between meals, so that by the time they eat their next supper, they're so hungry their resolve weakens and their choices spiral out of control. Snacking helps keep you satisfied and wards off cravings. And don't worry – it is supposed to feel a little indulgent.

Snacks don't have to be off-limits when eaten in moderation, and a variety of tasty and nutritious munchies can be included in a successful weight-loss program. In fact, choosing healthy snacks can help keep you from overeating later by satisfying hunger pains between meals. Fruits and vegetables can make you feel full in a hurry, even though they contain little fat and few calories. Fruits and vegetables contain fibre, minerals, vitamins and other nutrients. Whole-grain snacks such as crackers contain fibre and complex carbohydrates, which can increase your energy and stamina.

Protein-rich nuts and seeds can help you feel full until your next meal, but they are high in calories and also high in a healthy type of fat known as monounsaturated fat, so they should be eaten in moderation. Low-fat yogurt, cheese and other dairy products contain various vitamins and minerals while providing calcium and protein. The key is to focus on these kinds of healthy snacks when you need a little boost to tide you over before dinner time. Take them with a tall glass of water, which will help you feel full quickly, so at least you won't over-indulge and go overboard with this little snack break.

Healthy Snack Ideas

Two cups of carrots

One cup of sliced bananas or fresh berries

Two domino-sized slices of cheddar cheese

One cup of air-popped popcorn

An apple, an orange, a peach, a mango
or any other fruit

One-half cup of almonds or other nuts

Three whole-wheat crackers

A big glass of freshly squeezed fruit juice
(apple, orange, star fruit, etc.)

An unsweetened yogurt

One-half cup of dried raisins or dried cranberries

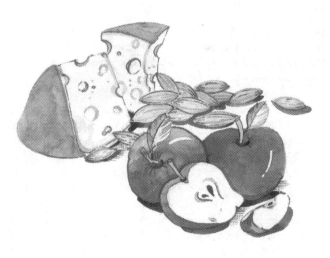

Drinks and Foods to Avoid

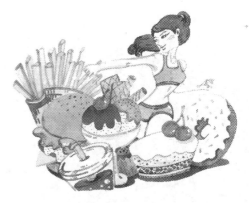

When dieting, beware of some foods and drinks which can secretly increase your calorie intake without your knowledge or notice. If you are not careful and continue to eat these kinds of foods, even in small portions, they will interfere with and may even halt your weight loss altogether. As mentioned in the previous chapters, your priority is to cut out a large part of your white starches or white carbohydrates. This means staying away from carbohydrates such as white rice, white pastas, breads, cakes and, to some extent, potatoes. White carbohydrates, sugar and fat are the most notorious food types for serious dieters. The high glycemic index of white carbohydrates increases glucose intake per portion. Moreover, this will amplify your appetite, compelling you to take additional food in between meals.

Here are the food groups which you need to avoid at all cost, or at least greatly limit if you want to succeed in your weight-loss endeavor:

Processed food – Say "NO" to any kind of processed food. The long shelf life of these foods is accomplished by adding preservatives. These preservatives are notorious for destabilizing the normal digestive process of your body.

Fast foods – This can easily invalidate the dieting process you are on. Almost all fast foods – or shall we call them "convenience foods" – are full of trans-fats and saturated fatty acids. As we consume them, they are broken down into cholesterol and glucose by several complex physiological processes in the liver. These products again transform the glucose and lipids to fat, only to be stored in the liver beneath the skin and other organs.

Colas or any sugary beverages – Sugary drinks are loaded with useless calories, and they have nothing else to offer. These kinds of drinks can only hamper your dieting. Drink lots of water in place of sugary or high-calorie beverages. Experiment with your water by adding lemon or cucumber for more flavor.

Alcohol – Alcohol counts as carbohydrates and as mentioned in a previous chapter, it can put your diet on hold. Give up alcohol while you diet or maybe indulge in a glass or two during your diet - pass meals.

Mayonnaise – A sandwich with mayonnaise sounds delicious, but mayonnaise contains saturated fatty acids in the form of oils and sugar. All these can greatly increase your total calorie intake and can once again make you lose control of your diet.

Avoid chocolate (or opt for dark chocolate only) – The high sugar and fat content can easily put chocolate away from your list of foods while dieting. A small piece of chocolate can give you instant energy if you are lethargic, but at the cost of high calories. Dark chocolate is a good alternative, and in general, you can expect fewer calories in it. Milk chocolates do have more calories because they have a higher percentage of sugar and milk vs. raw cocoa.

Avoid French fries and chips like the plague – Not only that, but every kind of deep - fried food should be avoided if you are dieting. They contain trans-fats and are loaded with calories, which puts you at a higher risk of heart disease. Restaurants like trans-fats since they make people feel satisfied quickly and allow cooks to use the same oil over and over again. The breading on fried food soaks up the grease. It's almost as bad as drinking oil straight from the vat.

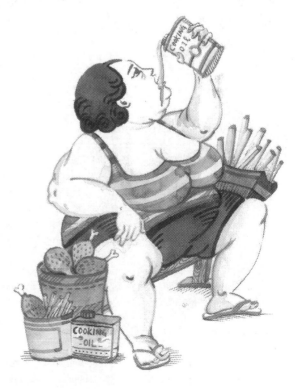

CHAPTER TWELVE

"THERE COMES A TIME IN EVERY WOMAN'S LIFE WHEN THE ONLY THING THAT HELPS IS A GLASS OF CHAMPAGNE."

BETTE DAVIS

Eating Foie Gras but Keeping It Real: Allowing Yourself a Few Indulgences And Balancing Eating Out with Your Diet

If you have ever been on a strict diet before, you know that as your body changes, your mind starts to play tricks on you. The longer you diet, the more you think about food until it becomes almost unbearable. It turns into an obsession and as you abstain, even the worst stuff begins to look good. My husband jokes that in some ways dieting is like sex – the longer you go without the "good stuff" (i.e. your favourite comfort foods), the crazier you get about them. And the mistake most people make at this point is to continue their strict diet, without giving themselves a little room to breath. This can sometimes lead to a mental breakdown or a large binge, and then as a result, some weight gain. When this happens, dieters often lose their resolve to continue and may at this crucial point even give up on the diet altogether.

Additionally, when you've been dieting for some time, you can also start feeling depressed, which is understandable, but not healthy. It is extremely important to take a break from dieting once in a while and have a "diet pass" at least a couple times a week. This means you can schedule about two meals a week during which you can eat some of your favourite foods (without binging). This will help take the edge off and keep you going. Nutrition experts will tell you that stopping and restarting your diet is sometimes the best way to bust through a weight plateau or to simply recharge your motivation.

That said, no one is telling you that a break from your diet is a free pass to start eating anything and everything you want. It certainly doesn't mean that you can go and buy a box of donuts, for instance, and proceed to consume all 12 in one go. A "diet pass" is a chance to relax and to stop being so vigilant for a little while. You should still eat smart and healthy, but you don't have to think about it for a certain stretch of time.

Having a special meal out with your partner or friends and ordering your favourite pasta, for instance, or even sharing the dessert you've been dreaming about is one way to enjoy what you have been yearning to eat. Pick a couple of meals a week (a dinner, a lunch or a breakfast) to indulge with that extra bit. Use that time to have what you've really been craving for – that way, you won't feel so frustrated. Try to remember the recommended ONE cupped-hand portion-control guideline for starches. Once again, the key is NOT to binge or to have too much of a setback with your diet. You don't want all that hard work to go to waste. This is just a little parenthesis in your diet, to help you keep your motivation strong and your mental state healthy and positive. In fact, eating in a disciplined way at home and enjoying yourself when you do eat out is the key to keeping your figure in check long term.

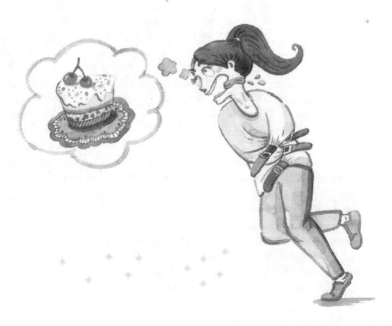

Whipping That Bootie Into Shape: The WORKOUT – Choose Your Cardio Workout The Importance of Increasing Your Metabolism

When it comes to weight loss, the importance of increasing your metabolism is paramount. This is the missing link that many of us do not think about. The calories you take in daily are regulated by your body's metabolism. How many are stored and how many are used are contingent upon increasing your metabolism. There is a simple way to look at this when it comes to how metabolism affects the goals you have for weight loss. The individual with a higher metabolism will either lose weight more rapidly or will not gain even if they eat the same amount as another person who has a slower metabolic rate. With all other factors constant, your metabolism can make a huge difference to how many and how fast you can lose those annoying pounds. So, here are some tips on increasing your metabolism to decrease your weight.

Include intense cardio and aerobic movements in your exercise regimen. If you want to increase your metabolism, make sure that you step up the aerobic exercises in your exercise regimen. Aerobic means "with oxygen," and refers to the use of oxygen in the body's metabolic or energy-generating process. Many types of exercises are aerobic, and by definition are performed at moderate levels of intensity for extended periods of time. An aerobic workout also helps you lose a lot of calories and can prove instrumental in helping you shed weight faster.

When asked about the benefits of boosting your metabolism, the immediate answer that most people give is: "I can eat more and lose weight faster." While it is true that an increase in your metabolism will result in you being able to consume more without necessarily gaining weight, it is not the only benefit. Boosting your metabolism means that you are going to be increasing the rate at which your body produces available energy. Think of your body as a factory which sometimes needs to be well oiled to function better and to help it access energy in a more efficient way. Your metabolism is basically the mechanism which your body uses to convert fat and calories into energy. Boosting your metabolism will mean that you suddenly will have an incredible increase in energy. Muscle tone will also improve, and your mental alertness will be amplified. When choosing a cardiovascular exercise program to boost your metabolism, you first need to consider three key elements: **how often, how long and how intensive** your workout should be.

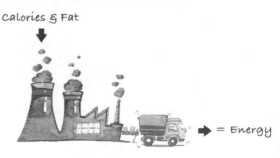

Calories & Fat

= Energy

How Often?

How often can you commit to exercising each week? In order to be efficient, you will need to commit to at least three or four sessions a week. In an ideal world, and for faster results, working out every day is recommended. Your body needs in some sense to be shaken from its "slumber" and put into high gear, so as to boost its metabolism quickly. It must get ready to access and burn all that additional energy which you have stored in your fat reserves during these long months of pregnancy. The real objective here is to quite literally "whip your bottom" into shape.

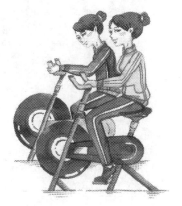

How Long?

For cardiovascular exercise to be effective, you will need a minimum of 20 to 30 minutes of nonstop exercise. Pick a pace that is sustainable for that amount of time which you will continue at an elevated but controlled heart rate. When you exercise, your body begins by first burning your stored carbohydrates, but as the workout continues, it will tap into your stored fats for more energy and fuel. This moment is crucial for your weight loss and often called the "fat-burning" stage. And when you feel tired towards the middle or end of your cardio workout, think of this actually taking place in your body. "Feel the burn" and keep going till your target workout time has been reached.

You need to push your body steadily to help it increase its metabolism. Nonetheless, it is important that you listen to your body and not go overboard. You will know when you are ready to increase or even sometimes decrease your workout depending on how you feel each day. If you've had a terrible night's sleep, go for a shorter or more moderate workout that day. If you feel strong and energized, try to extend your workout by 10 or 15 minutes. The key is to be flexible, but to try to hit that minimum weekly workout routine.

How Intensive?

What is the right level of intensity? There are a number or cardio options for your workout, so how do you know you've picked one with the right level of intensity? You know you are working out at the right level when it is difficult to carry on a conversation while exercising. We are not taking a stroll in the park here, girls! We are excercising. The goal is to build your endurance and strength, and depending on what level you've picked on a machine or what cardio workout you've chosen outdoors, the emphasis should be on the workout being challenging but achievable. Selecting the type of exercise is the key. Remember you will need to opt for one that will elevate your heart rate.

Once you have chosen a cardio program that works for you - you may also decide to combine several cardio options instead of sticking to just one - the important part is to fully commit yourself to the process. This is the only way you will get lasting results. While it is important to listen to your body, the workout still needs to push your limits. And it may at times feel tiring and uncomfortable, but you must persevere.

To get the body you dream of, only YOU can make it happen. Look at a woman in the gym whose body you admire – trust me, she didn't get it just because she was born that way. There is no secret. She looks this way because she has worked hard at her fitness and has made calculated choices with her nutrition.

When you decide to go for a workout, it needs to count. Putting on your gym outfit and walking into the gym and stetching is not enough. You need to come out of that workout session sweating and panting. Your 20, 30 or 40 minutes of cardio workout is serious business. It's not a social event that lets you chat with your friends. You need to stay focused and get it done. It should become a part of your life, a routine if you will. And if you are using machines at a gym and looking at how many calories you burn during your workout, burning about 250, 350 or 400 calories per workout is enough, especially given you are also dieting and controlling your food intake. And if you stick to this exercise routine once you have reached your ideal weight, you will be able to eat more moderately and never worry about putting on weight in the future.

You must also remember that while we all have our personal limitations, constraints and different body types with genetic predispositions, we can still strive to have the best body we possibly can. Fitting in a fat-burning cardio workout several times a week into your busy schedule will have its numerous rewards. Not only will you be able to lose the extra pounds and reach your target weight, but you will also feel better and more confident about yourself. Working out gives you more energy throughout the day; it increases the quality of your sleep and your overall health. So keep pushing yourself. Make fitting your workout in your schedule a priority. And when exercising outdoors or at the gym, be sure to get the MOST out of your workout routine.

Cardio Options

Jogging (one of the highest calorie burners)

Brisk Walking

Spinning

Jumping Rope

Bicycling

Tennis

Squash

Swimming

Rowing

Dancing

Aerobics

Stepping

Skiing

Rollerblading

Roller Skating

Ice Skating

Kickboxing

Nordic Track Elliptical Machine

Stair Climbing or Stair Master

Zumba

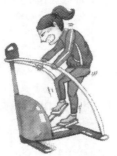

Swear Master

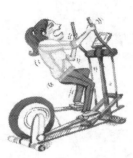

Nordic Trick

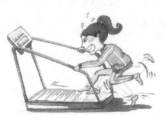

Dread Mill

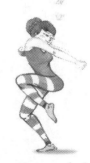

Zumba Draining

Weekly Cardio Schedule Sample

Different types of cardiovascular exercises can be combined to make your workout more enjoyable and exciting. If you prefer to stick to one, that's also fine, but I highly recommend you combine at least two or three different types every week. Don't forget to do basic stretches before you begin, so as to improve your flexibility, which in turn may improve your athletic performance and decrease your risk of injury.

LIGHT WORKOUT OPTION – Brisk walking, biking and Nordic track elliptical

Monday	Tuesday	Wednesday	Thursday	Friday	Saturday	Sunday
	5-7 minutes basic stretching		5-7 minutes basic stretching		5-7 minutes basic stretching	
	35-40 minutes brisk walking		20 minutes Nordic track elliptical		25-30 minutes biking	

MORE INTENSE WORKOUT OPTION- Zumba, jogging and swimming

Monday	Tuesday	Wednesday	Thursday	Friday	Saturday	Sunday
5-7 minutes basic stretching		5-7 minutes basic stretching		5-7 minutes basic stretching		5-7 minutes basic stretching
20-25 minutes jogging		45 minute to 1 hour Zumba dance class		20-25 minutes jogging		30 minutes swimming
15 minutes biking				15 minutes biking		

CHAPTER FOURTEEN

"I HAVE GAINED AND LOST THE SAME TEN POUNDS SO MANY TIMES OVER AND OVER AGAIN, MY CELLULITE MUST HAVE DÉJÀ VU."

JANE WAGNER

Banishing Cottage Cheese Thighs:
The All Out War on Cellulite

When working hard to get your figure and especially your derrière in the best post-pregnancy-shape possible, cellulite is the enemy. The truth is, you don't even have to be overweight to have cellulite. Thin people can suffer from it too. I was lucky enough to be invited and had front row tickets to a lingerie show ONCE. There were lots of leggy models strutting down the runway, but there was one thing that made me cringe in my chair (you do know why I have this particular phobia) - several of these young models had bad cellulite. At first I thought it was the lighting. Was it the angle at which I was watching them from? Was it something in my cocktail? Finally I realized that these skinny ladies - gasp! - just happened to have bad cellulite, probably from poor eating habits and not enough exercise.

A lot of people suffer from cellulite, a toxic build-up manifested by orange peel skin and cottage cheese thighs. Cellulite is different from regular fat, which is smoother to the touch when squeezed. Regular fat is held in place by a network of fibres, and when the system works well, all waste products are removed from this system resulting in smooth body curves. When the waste removal system stars to fail, waste products build up and the connective tissue becomes saturated with liquid, which then thickens and hardens – forming small hard pockets that puff up to produce the "orange peel" or "cottage cheese" effect.

Many factors can contribute to having cellulite such as insufficient water intake, little or no exercise, constipation and digestion problems, stress, fatigue, hormonal cycles, excess weight, pollution and poor diet. And when a woman is pregnant, her body is flooded with estrogen which causes her to store more fat so that she may have sufficient calories available for lactation post delivery. This is why most women who've had children may notice more cellulite on their thighs and bottom after pregnancy.

The main remedy for fighting cellulite is to detoxify the body. Getting rid of cellulite needs dedication and consistent work. Regular fat can be found anywhere on the body but cellulite tends to settle on the following areas: the back of the thighs, buttocks, hips and stomach, which is where women tend to store the biggest percentage of their body fat. Breastfeeding can help greatly reduce water retention and cellulite post pregnancy, but to banish cellulite in the long run, only diet and exercise really work in my opinion. Cellulite is thought to occur in 80 to 90% of post pubescent females and most women have some amount of cellulite no matter how fit they are. The key is to banish it or at least minimize it as much as possible. I can say from a personal standpoint that I have less cellulite now than I did when I was 25 years old. At that time I was taking birth control pills (which can lead to water retention) and was less disciplined with my exercise and diet regime. After having my first child, I decided that I was going to make my fitness a big priority in my life. So I started the **Mummylicious** diet and workout program, and as I improved my lifestyle, I minimized my cellulite. Many women wonder if cellulite can really go away with diet and exercise. The answer to this question is yes. Aerobic exercise has been proven to be the best kind of exercise to reduce cellulite long term. Cellulite is mainly caused by poor blood circulation in the body, so cardiovascular exercise stimulates the blood and lymphatic circulation. By jogging or biking for example, the body sweat detoxifies the skin and burns body fat. And as you build more muscles from regular exercise, it will also give you more muscular definition which tends to make cellulite less visible.

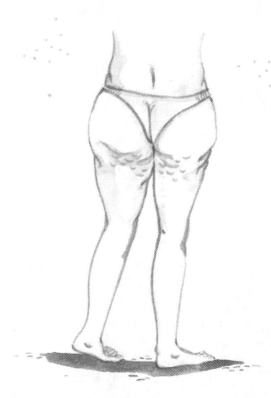

So what else can you do to fight cellulite? Honestly, not much more. By combining a healthy diet with periods of ketosis, and a regular fat burning cardiovascular exercise program, you are fighting cellulite naturally. What you CAN do, if you still want to further try to reduce the appearance of cellulite and help detoxify your body, are the following three things:

1. Powerful Cellulite Massage - When the skin is firmly massaged, the blood flow increases as well as does the lymphatic drainage - the result of which is the reduction of fluid in the dermis area and a lessening of cellulite. This cellulite reduction can be easily seen when problem areas on the skin begin to become less bloated and puffy. This technique cannot remove cellulite completely, but may have a temporary effect in reducing the amount of "dimpling" appearance. Unfortunately, specialized cellulite massage cannot be done by anyone at any time, as it takes a specific method to achieve the desired results. To be truly effective, lymphatic massage should be performed by a specialist. But in the absence of a trained professional, a vigorous Swedish massage is also greatly beneficial.

2. Water Consumption - This natural way of getting rid of cellulite requires only that you drink more water. Water is a natural cleanser and detoxifier, that can help repair the connective tissue in your body, thereby making it harder for cellulite to accumulate. So drink as much water as you can, at least 8 to 10 glasses a day and more if you are exercising.

3. Natural Anti-Cellulite Creams – There is no proven, effective topical method that gets rid of cellulite, but there are numerous creams & lotion on the market that claim they can visibly help in reducing its look and feel. The important thing to remember when buying anti-cellulite creams is the content. It does no good to buy creams if all they really do is moisturize the skin and temporarily improve appearances. You need to know what ingredients are contained within the cream and if those ingredients are in any way effective in the treatment of cellulite. So, what ingredients should you look for in a cellulite cream? There are really only two main ones you need to worry about:

Caffeine is probably the most common ingredient you will find in cellulite lotion. Caffeine is a stimulant and a vasodilator, which means it opens up blood vessels and helps to reduce fat cells. It can enhance fat metabolism and also reduce some of the edema, or swelling that we get around the fat, so the skin appears smoother.

Aminophylline is actually a drug that is used to treat asthma. When applied topically, it works to dehydrate the skin by eliminating excess water and thus reduces the appearance of cellulite. The affected areas appear smoother and more firm but it's sort of like taking a diuretic to lose weight – so it's not really fat that you're losing, but rather water.

While cellulite creams and massages may help to some extent, by improving the appearance of your skin, in my view they are far less efficient than a healthy diet and regular exercise in winning the war against cellulite. To be effective, the creams would have to be used in sufficient quantities for a prolonged period of time. However, studies have shown a small reduction in thigh girth when using these creams, yet not a substantial change in cellulite. Ultimately I only see one real and bona fide solution to minimizing cellulite - diet and exercise. Several studies have proven that female athletes, who generally have a lower percent of body fat, have less cellulite than most women. Thus you can safely conclude that if you combine aerobic exercise with a calorie-restricted diet plan, such as the one recommended in this book, it will greatly help in reducing your underlying body fat reserves, and further lessen your cellulite to give you the most promising and realistic results.

CHAPTER FIFTEEN

"MUSIC WASHES AWAY FROM THE SOUL THE DUST OF EVERYDAY LIFE."

BERTHOLD AUERBACH

Feel the Beat:
Benefits of Music for Your Cardio Workouts

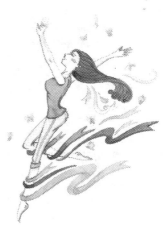

Music is a brilliant way to energize the body by way of your cardio workout. Adding music to your exercise routine will greatly increase the intensity level, plus it will make it more fun and effortless. It has been proven to help you exercise better and longer. But there are many other benefits to adding music to your workout, such as increased focus and motivation. Music can also make you feel like you're not working as hard as you really are. Repetitive exercises can be boring, so listening to music while you exercise will help remove this boredom and as a result help you commit to putting more effort into your workout. Because it makes you feel happier, it can give you a boost to keep moving even if you're tired or uncomfortable. If you match the beat of the music to your workout, it can improve the pace of your movements – while keeping you working out longer. Exercising to music helps you be "in the moment" – keeping your mind focused on your movements, so you can carry on moving at a steady pace.

On the days when I don't feel like working out, I go to the gym anyway and simply start walking on the treadmill listening to my music. Oftentimes, 15 minutes into my walk, I am so uplifted and relaxed by the music that I suddenly feel like jogging and increasing my pace. Music has the power to make you want to move, to jog, to dance and even sing. It leads you to find the energy you didn't think you had. Listening to music on your way to the gym also puts you in the mood to work out, because an important part of working out is being in the right positive and energized mental state.

What type of music should you work out to? That's up to you. Pick what's fun, but also think about trying to match the beat to whatever physical activity you've chosen. Studies show that most people say they feel that music helps them make their exercise more enjoyable. It seems clear that music makes people like exercise better and helps them feel better exercising. This means that if you work out to music, you're probably going to have a good time. And as a result, you'll be more likely to keep up with your exercise and exercise longer than without music.

Additionally, not only can listening to music reduce depression, stress and anxiety, but it can also relieve pain. Music has been proven to help the body release endorphins, which are small protein molecules that are produced by the nervous system and other parts of your body. An important role of endorphins is to work with sedative receptors that are known to relieve common pain. These analgesia-producing receptors are located in your brain, spinal cord and other nerve endings. As endorphins are released in your body when you listen to music, the obvious benefits will be to make a tough workout more bearable and thus more enjoyable.

Creating a playlist of all your favourite danceable tunes and high-impact beats for your workout is a hugely motivational factor when finding the willpower to go to the gym. Music puts you in a good mood, and when you are involved in an activity that is enjoyable you will want to repeat and continue that activity in the future. The reverse is also true. If an action is rewarded with a negative feeling or experience, that action will come across as unpleasant and as a result this increases the chances of it not being repeated. Combining the pleasure of music with physical exercise is more likely to result in you continuing your exercise routine with greater motivation and discipline.

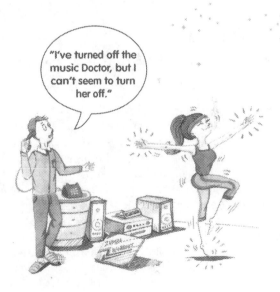

CHAPTER SIXTEEN

"FOCUSING ON THE ACT OF BREATHING CLEARS THE MIND OF ALL DAILY DISTRACTIONS AND CLEARS OUR ENERGY, ENABLING US TO BETTER CONNECT WITH THE SPIRIT WITHIN."

AUTHOR UNKNOWN

In and Out?
Breathing RIGHT While You Exercise

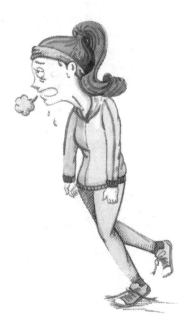

Depending on the type of cardio exercise you choose and on the level of intensity, breathing can become the key to whether or not you succeed in reaching your own workout objectives. Sometimes people can't finish their workout because they run out of breath and have to stop. Instead, it is better to start out by being aware of how you breathe, and to make your breath the primary focus. The best way to remember how to breathe during a workout is to control your breathing. Many people end up exercising very intensely to the point where they have to stop in order to catch their breath. It is better to remain aware of your breathing at all times and to focus on controlling how you breathe. You don't want to be huffing and puffing loudly while you exercise. If you find it difficult to catch your breath, this probably means that you need to lower the intensity of your workout and build on from there.

In some sports such as marital arts, breathing is often the focus because it allows the body to maximize the oxygen that reaches the muscles and keeps the energy levels high. By focusing your attention on a specific and repetitive movement, the mind can become immersed in the moment; as a result, the person can exercise much longer and more comfortably because their attention is not focused on how tired they feel. Controlling your breathing can help you channel your mind while you exercise. It allows you to think about other things in your life, to refocus your energy on your daily goals. This form of meditation can help sharpen your resolve to reach your objectives and increases your focus on the task at hand. Even with dance music's repetitive beat, your controlled breathing combined with the regular movements of your exercise routine, can lead you into a trance-like meditative state.

Breathing technique is also very important. In general, when exercising, try to breathe in through the nose and exhale through the mouth. This way, you remain focused on your breathing without becoming focused on how out of breath you are. Some people often disregard this technique and ultimately experience side stitches and cramps. This is because your body needs a sufficient amount of oxygen to maintain your tempo, keep you focused and make your training more efficient. The stronger the exercise, the deeper you need to breathe. Avoid shallow breaths which allow carbon dioxide to accumulate in your body and which also result in decreasing your physical endurance.

Therefore, while doing cardio exercises such as jogging, biking or even brisk walking, you need to breathe in deeper to ensure your body gets enough oxygen. Never hold your breath; make sure you are establishing an inhale/exhale pattern that is comfortable for you and suitable for the activity. And while it is advisable to breathe in through your nose and exhale through your mouth, it is also important to take your own personal needs into consideration. Some people may find it difficult to nose breathe and may prefer to breathe in and out through the mouth during intense cardio exercise. It is vital to pay attention to your own body's needs and to find a breathing technique that you are comfortable with. The key is to ensure your body gets enough oxygen while exercising. In time and by trying different ways of breathing, you can find a healthy and effective method that allows for overall optimum athletic performance.

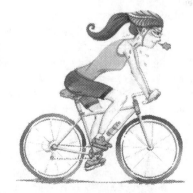

CHAPTER SEVENTEEN

"PHYSICAL FITNESS IS THE FIRST REQUISITE OF HAPPINESS."
JOSEPH H. PILATES

Flat Abs, a Tighter Tush and Killer Legs: Benefits of Pilates for Post-Delivery Bodies

Have you ever tried doing a sit-up a few months after giving birth? Well, I did.

Let me tell you, as sad as it is to admit it, I did not even manage to lift my upper torso one inch off the floor! That's right – ZERO muscle tone on my tummy. I felt like a sea cucumber, only fatter and more limp. This is completely normal, given that our abdominal muscles after pregnancy are still in the recovery mode. Under the influence of the relaxin hormone, they undergo a dramatic change and a tremendous amount of stretching in all directions. Connective tissues within the muscles provide a degree of elasticity, but the main transformation occurs in the connective tissues joining the transversal and oblique abdominal muscles. These abdominal muscles, which at first lay parallel on your tummy, stretch away gradually as the pregnancy progresses and eventually separate from the mid-line, to allow more space for the growing uterus. As it is not painful, many women will be unaware that this has happened, although they may experience chronic backache as a result.

Pilates, a form of exercise developed by Joseph Pilates during the 1920s in Germany, is a wonderful solution for mums who want to strengthen and reshape their bodies after pregnancy. It is designed to fortify abdominal core muscles, improve muscle control, and emphasizes the balanced development of the body through core rebuilding and flexibility. Naturally, before signing up for any such classes, make sure that your body and your muscles have completely healed after the birth.

It is generally advisable to wait a minimum of three months after delivery to start a postnatal Pilates class. If you've had a C-section, however, then it is highly recommended that you wait a minimum of five to six months before starting. Once more, I cannot stress enough how important it is to check in with your doctor before beginning any kind of postnatal exercise or exercise class.

The Pilates program you choose should be designed to suit your individual post-delivery needs. Every woman has a different and unique experience of pregnancy, birth and how she feels thereafter. Done under qualified instruction, Pilates can also help women who have experienced birth complications recover more quickly. The breathing technique used in Pilates increases oxygen and blood flow, which both aid the healing process. But in the end, Pilates still offers one of the best methods to get back into stronger shape quickly after having a baby. By committing to as little as an hour-long weekly exercise session, you will be able to see results straight away. The benefits of postnatal Pilates classes are numerous. Designed specifically to target those problem areas that mothers face after pregnancy, these classes are conceived to firm up and strengthen the body's core muscles in order to create a trimmer and sleeker silhouette. By creating a "muscle girdle" around your middle, you will have greater strength in your back and stomach muscles, while also improving your posture and reducing your back pain, especially if you are still breastfeeding. In the meantime, and if you are up for it, while waiting to join a proper Pilates class, you can also start with three simple Pilates floor exercises which you can perform at home. If you don't have a Pilates mat, find a rug or a carpeted area in your home, where you can try the following muscle-strengthening movements at your own pace and leisure.

Three Simple Pilates Mat Exercises Which You Can Start at Home

The Hundred – Good for strengthening abdominal muscles

Start by lying on your back with your legs straight. Lift the legs at a 45-degree angle or higher if your stomach muscles are not yet strong enough. Bring your head up with your chin down, and lift your shoulder blades off the floor. Pull your abdomen in toward your spine and lift the arms about four inches off the ground. Each cycle is five short in-breaths and then five short out-breaths (like sniffing in and puffing out). Continue until you complete 10 sets, which equals 100 total seconds. Lower your legs and return to your starting position.

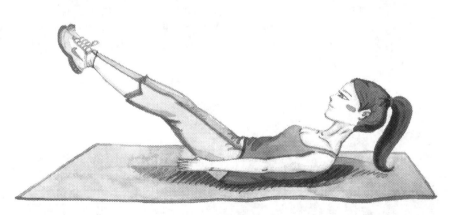

Swimming - Good for strengthening and lengthening the back muscles

Start by lying on your stomach with your arms outstretched above your head. Take a deep breath in, and then breath out as you lift your right arm and left leg two inches off the ground, stretching the arm and leg as you lift. Lower the arm and leg and repeat on the opposite side with the left arm and right leg. You can start with slow repetitions, and then increase in speed. Complete eight repetitions, rest and then perform two additional sets. Hopefully you will feel like you are simulating swimming!

Leg Circles - Good for loosening tight hips and strengthening legs and abdominal muscles

Start by lying on your back with your legs straight. Pull one of your knees in toward your chest and open the leg up. Circle it outward and back in to your starting position. Repeat this until you have completed eight circles and alternate with the other leg. Rest, and then perform an additional set of circles one leg at a time. You may choose to do this exercise with one leg, or both legs at the same time (which is more difficult).

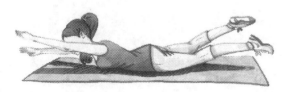

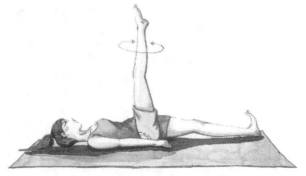

CHAPTER EIGHTEEN

"I'M BRINGIN' SEXY BACK."

JUSTIN TIMBERLAKE

The Finish Line and Getting Your Body Back: Maintaining Your Figure – A Lifetime Commitment

Combining regular cardio exercises and ideally a weekly Pilates class, plus a low-carbohydrate and portion-control diet should almost assuredly get you to your target weight. Once you've reached your goal and have succeeded in strengthening and toning up your body after delivery, you will feel an enormous sense of achievement. You should be very proud of yourself, and you must absolutely celebrate this big accomplishment. The road less travelled is what you have chosen, and every bit of effort and all the sacrifices you've made along the way are worth the reward of how you feel and look today. You may even notice that you walk with a new spring in your step, having more confidence and self-esteem in your heart. Savour your moment of success, but don't simply rest on your laurels.

What comes next, now that you have reached your goal? Maintaining your figure is a lifetime commitment. The key is to continue with your sports activities and to keep a tight control on your food intake. It's simple: if you suddenly stop exercising and start eating too much, you will put all the weight back on – there is no secret here. This is usually the problem for many women who feel very motivated to diet and exercise soon after having a baby, but as the months and years go by, the discipline slowly dies out and the pounds start to pile back on. You have a full life to live and enjoy, so hang on to this feeling of pure satisfaction. Now that you are at your ideal weight, commit to sustaining it for the foreseeable future, by showing flexible restraint in your approach to food and by keeping regular exercise in your weekly schedule.

Rather than following a rigid all-or-nothing rule, keep making healthy choices. No foods should be seen as completely forbidden. This means enjoying small amounts of favourite foods without feeling guilty. And if you do over-indulge or have a big night out, cut back the next day, or have a longer workout to balance things out.

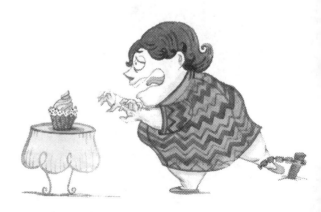

Learning how to choose, prepare and enjoy a balanced diet, as well as understanding food labels and having the ability to judge portion sizes, are important skills in helping you stick to your ideal weight long term. Eating regular meals, taking time to really taste them and allowing yourself to indulge on occasion are all part of a healthy attitude towards food. Continue to eat a balanced, lower fat diet with plenty of fruit and vegetables. Don't avoid any food, just watch portion sizes (remember the ONE cupped-hand portion guide for starches) and limit the amount of certain fatty foods. When bringing more carbohydrates back into your diet, be sure to choose whole-grain rice, pastas and breads if you can (as they contain more fibre and nutrients than the regular kind). Have three regular meals a day at set times and small snacks on occasion. Eat out once in a while, but stay away from fast food. Sit down to eat your meals. Take time over them and pay attention to what you're eating. Keep "self-monitoring" to stay conscious of your new eating and activity habits. For many people, food is a quick and effective way to deal with stress. If this sounds like you, take some time to reflect on the stresses in your life and how you respond to them. Think about how you can manage stress differently.

Most importantly, remember that getting regular exercise is one of the strongest indicators of long-term success. Even as little as 30 minutes three or four times a week will be enough to keep your metabolism up. And not only does it help burn calories and keep your muscles strong, exercise will also boost your self-esteem and decrease your stress levels.

As we get older, our metabolism slows down, and it becomes much easier to gain weight and get out of shape fast. The older you get, the tougher it is to lose weight, because by then, your body and your fat are really "good friends." It takes serious effort and commitment to maintain your weight and stay in shape all your life. It's something you have to want to work hard at and be willing to adjust to in the long term. Once you find a good balance between watching your diet and sticking to a regular exercise routine, you will see that maintaining your figure and health will become second nature. It will simply develop into another important priority in your life, alongside caring for your children and your family.

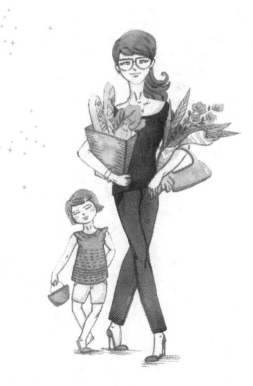

A Few Tricks that Work

Drink at least eight or ten glasses of water a day.
Have a big glass of water before meals and especially if you are very hungry.

Skip desserts, especially at night.
Have a piece of black chocolate instead if you crave something sweet.

Don't eat your dinner too late or too close to your bedtime.
Ideally, dine at least four hours before you sleep at night.

Drink green tea occasionally so as to help boost your metabolism.
Green tea also promotes fat oxidation.

Eat slowly and chew your food well before swallowing.
This seems basic, but we often eat too fast and as a result too much.

Develop the habit of weighing yourself everyday or every other day, to keep a close watch on your weight.
It may seem excessive, but it's a good habit to keep you vigilant with your weight.

Try having a couple of big glasses of fruit or vegetable juice instead of dinner on Sunday nights, especially if you've had a big weekend of eating and drinking.
Try an apple, carrot and celery combo in a juicer - it's delicious.

Get a Doggie Bag if you can.
Most restaurants in Europe don't allow it, but if you live in a country that does, by all means you don't have to overeat – take it home!

Limit your salt.
Excess sodium intake can lead to water retention and hypertension.

Whenever possible, switch to whole grain rice, bread, pastas which are richer in nutrients and fibre than refined starches.

As much as possible, stick to grilled, baked or roasted meats, chicken and fish.
Avoid eating fried, breaded or deep-fried food.

Stop eating before you are full.
It takes time for the signal to reach your brain that you've had enough. Avoid the temptation to clean your plate.

Go easy on the booze.
Advice I admit I don't always follow myself.

Out of sight, out of mind – limit the amount of tempting foods you have at home.
Store snack foods and other high-calorie indulgences in cabinets out of your sight.

Get your partner to join your diet and exercise program.
Doing this as a team is always more motivational.

Get plenty of sleep.
Lack of sleep has been shown to have a direct link to hunger, overeating and weight gain. Exhaustion also impairs your judgment, which can lead to poor food choices. Aim for around eight hours of quality sleep a night.

Lastly, when tempted to have a second serving, remember: it's not your LAST meal!
You can always eat more tomorrow.

CHAPTER NINETEEN

"THE ONE THING THAT MATTERS IS THE EFFORT."

ANTOINE DE SAINT-EXUPERY

Frump Mummy Is OUT – Mummylicious Is IN: The Importance of Grooming And Making an Effort to Dress and Look Your Best

Having a new baby can be overwhelming for any new mum. Especially if it's your first child. It's easy to get lost in the responsibility of a new family because for the first time in your life, you now have to put this tiny little helpless being first, even before your own basic needs. Often we focus so hard on our new baby that our own essential grooming and dressing standards quickly go out the window. But I tell you, children grow up fast, become very independent, and if you are not careful as the years go by, you're left standing with bad hair, a big belly, a saggy bottom and no sense of style to speak of.

Despite the difficult time constraints a new mother may have, being at least clean and well-groomed should be the bare minimum. As essential and as basic as it seems, this first step can often be compromised. No matter how busy you may be, this is the prerequisite that you absolutely need to uphold. Showering every day and washing your hair at least every couple of days is a must. If you don't have time for regular manicures and pedicures, keep your nails short and clean. This applies to your hair, too. Forget high-maintenance hairdos – keep your hairstyle simple and neat, easy to wash and arrange. Don't forget to shave your legs and underarms, and pluck your eyebrows, too. If you don't have time for a bikini wax, keep it nice and trim down below. You certainly don't want to frighten your partner with a wild and out of control jungle south of the border!

In terms of dressing, it's not about having a big wardrobe or a multitude of choices, but rather sticking to the styles and colours that flatter you most and that suit your lifestyle. If you are still nursing, you will be more restricted in the type and cut of your outfits. Be practical with your dressing choices. As Coco Chanel once declared, "Being elegant does not consist of putting on a new dress." Elegance, in my view, comes from simplicity and from being well-groomed. Taking pride in your appearance should not be limited to being physically fit. It also means you make the effort to dress and look your very best.

If you really don't have time for much make-up, just try a quick touch of mascara or a little blush on your cheeks. It will give you that extra glow and will make you feel more attractive and confident. And let's face it, the most beautiful thing a woman can ever wear is not an expensive designer outfit – it's her confidence. And in truth, she is never as attractive as when she has the belief that she is beautiful.

All these little efforts in your appearance – be it with your dress, your accessories or your make-up – will go a long way to make you feel more feminine and attractive. You won't be doing it just for your partner or for your family and friends – you will be doing it for yourself. And it's not about wearing stilettos to a school picnic, but about remaining practical, yet always with a certain pride in your overall appearance. Being **Mummylicious** is in fact simply wanting to look great. It goes hand in hand with your desire to be fit and healthy, and it means you aspire to feel proud of yourself, too.

We sometimes see mums on the street who seem to have given up on their appearance altogether. It's as if the moment they became mothers, they stopped caring about their figure and their looks. They sometimes seem as if they make no effort to dress or even appear well groomed. And lets be honest, we've all had "moments" when we've found ourselves so completely overwhelmed with having a new baby that our appearance, temporarily, takes a back seat. But in the long term, no amount of excuses, can justify letting yourself go entirely and giving up on yourself in this way.

Motherhood does not have to mean the end of your most feminine and attractive years. You don't have to become the stereotype of a frumpy mummy if you don't want to be. And remember sometimes – it's not just who you are that holds you back, but also who you think you cannot be. At the end of the day, it all depends on your own desire to succeed. If you WANT to be **Mummylicious**, you must believe in your heart that you can be just that. You can be the very best you can possibly be if you truly wish it and act on it. Because in essence, I am convinced that there is no such thing as an ugly woman, but – to put it very frankly – just a lazy one.

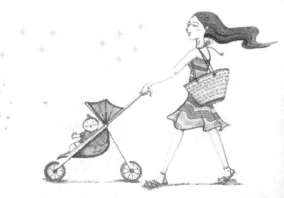

And Finally...

> "THE AIM OF LIFE IS SELF-DEVELOPMENT. TO REALIZE ONE'S NATURE PERFECTLY – THAT IS WHAT EACH OF US IS HERE FOR."
>
> OSCAR WILDE

And Finally...On Getting Your Groove Back and Being Mummylicious: Don't Focus Just On Your Looks – Cultivate Your Mind

Getting your groove back after having a baby is no easy mission. Some women never get "it" back. The "it" here refers to their past sexiness, their youthful lusciousness, their energy and joie de vivre and especially their figure. Some women become so overwhelmed with the shock to the system of having a baby that they completely "lose" themselves in the whole miracle of becoming a parent. Their lifestyle changes so drastically, sleep deprivation hits hard, priorities change – the baby MUST come first. It takes a certain strength of character to say "STOP! Wait! I'm still here! I'm still the same woman but better, stronger, more experienced!" Getting your groove back is an uphill battle which begins the moment your get home from the hospital.

You first need to reorganize your life around this new baby. Then as time passes, you slowly need to find a way to re-conquer your body. Getting your groove back starts with getting your body back.

And remember, getting your body back often leads to having a better sex life, too. But what about your mind? Don't forget that important part of you. Some say that delivering your baby is like delivering your brains. I will tell you that my memory was never as bad as when I was sleep-deprived and breastfeeding these four kids. It's so easy to lose your sense of self, your desire to dress, your ambition, your passion for life and your craving to learn anything new. For a lot of mums, the first year of having a baby seems like a blur, but when the dust finally settles, what's left of you?

If you don't make your well-being one of your priorities in life, your self-esteem may eventually hit rock bottom and you may even risk sliding into depression. Choosing to be **Mummylicious** can help you give yourself that fundamental and critical importance. And being **Mummylicious** doesn't mean you are trying to be perfect – no one is. It simply means that now that you are a mummy, and especially because you are a mummy, you have committed to always trying to look and be your very best. No more excuses. Being **Mummylicious** is not just about being fit – it's an attitude to life. As I like to think:

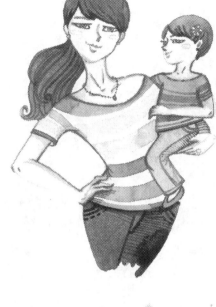

"I'm a mother and I'm proud of it.
But I'm still, first and foremost, a woman.
I'm not past my prime after having a baby.
I feel more beautiful and
more confident than ever."

You must believe with a strong conviction that a woman can be more attractive after having a baby, and you don't have to be a conventional beauty at all. It just takes a little more effort and discipline, for most of us, to re-conquer our figure and strengthen and heal our bodies after having a baby. Being beautiful and feeling sexy are easier when you feel good about your figure, of course, but it's not nearly enough. You need to look at all aspects of your life and try to balance those parts, too.

Do you have your own convictions, beliefs you stick to? Do you take care of yourself not just physically, but also emotionally and mentally? If you are planning to go back to work or work part-time, is it a career choice that is worth, in your mind, spending so much time away from your child? Is your job making your happy? If you have decided not to go back to work, do you have an interesting hobby – something in your life unrelated to your children? It can be anything from a charity you feel passionate about, to a course you've always wanted to take, to starting a book club among friends, learning a new craft, setting up a small internet business or even writing a book - anything, really.

As the American novelist Henry Miller counseled: "Develop interest in life as you see it; in people, things, literature, music – the world is so rich, simply throbbing with rich treasures, beautiful souls and interesting people." There are many facets in your life that need attention. But being physically fit after having a baby is a strong first step in that direction. Being self-disciplined and exercising the willpower to attain your fitness goals is just the start. Once you succeed, the sense of achievement and pride cannot be underestimated. It shows you care enough about yourself to take the time and energy to look your very best.

Every woman who becomes a mother needs to think about what will make her feel truly fulfilled in the future. Being a mother is a privilege and a great responsibility, but is it enough? If you love and respect yourself, you will make it a priority to take care of all the other important aspects of your life. And cultivating your mind is a big part of being fulfilled.

The friends you choose will also have a big influence on your life. Support is extremely important for any new mum. Choose to be around women you admire, who inspire you and whom you can learn from. As my mother often wisely says, "Don't waste time with people who don't enhance your life." Stay away from negative people who will bring you down and suck your precious energy. As a mother, you have to be more selective, organized and productive with your time. Every minute of your day counts!

For the long term and for your own future well-being, find a way to invest time and energy in an interest that cultivates your intellect. If you develop a passion for learning, you will never cease to grow, and true fulfillment comes from that. As the children get older and become more independent, it will give you something to fall back on and in many ways it will make you feel more confident and accomplished.

Real beauty is derived from believing in yourself and knowing that you are capable of achieving anything you set your mind to. Great strength comes from the determination to follow your own path in life and from not being easily thrown off by obstacles along the way. Ultimately, it's about self-respect, one of the most important and key attributes to feeling attractive inside and out. Every woman can emit positive and confident energy and her own unique brand of sexiness. The great screen siren Sophia Loren once declared that "sex appeal is 50% what you've got, and 50% what other people think you've got." And this attitude, in my opinion, embodies exactly what it truly means to be **Mummylicious**. So mark my words, ladies, and watch out, because **Mummyliciousness** is contagious!

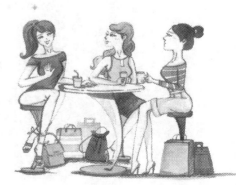

THE MUMMYLICIOUS CHECKLIST

Top FIVE Things on the Mummylicious Checklist

01. Make time to exercise regularly – commit to at least three or four times a week.

02. Watch what you eat. Think about everything you put into your body.

03. Monitor your weight carefully. It should become a reflex to help you calibrate your food intake and your exercise routine and intensity.

04. Always make an effort to be well-groomed and to dress and look your best.

05. Cultivate your mind and never stop learning.

THE MUMMYLICIOUS
PROGRESS TABLE

Date					
Weight					
Breasts					
Waist					
Hips					
Thighs					

THE MUMMYLICIOUS
WEIGHT-LOSS CONTRACT

I, ..., on this date, ..., being of sound mental health and possessed of full mental capacity, hereby agree and commit to reaching my target weight of .... by the following date ....

Monthly Target Weight-Loss Objective:.........................

Halfway Mark Target-Weight Objective: This weight.................. by this date: ....

Ideal Target Body Measurements: .... (Breasts) - .... (Waist) - .... (Hips) - .... (Thighs)

The reasons I want to lose weight and get my figure back are:..
....
....

Some of the other benefits of reaching my goals are:..
....
....

ACTION PLAN:

I commit to taking the following steps to improve my accountability to myself and increase my chances for weight-loss success:

1. I promise to find the time to exercise at least............... times a week for at least............... minutes.

2. The type of exercise/sport I plan to do: ....
....
....

How will I alternate them on which days and for how long each etc...(be specific): ....
....

3. I promise to refrain from eating the following foods until I reach my goal: ....
....

(except when I have a pre-organized "diet-pass" meal, which I will enjoy without bingeing)

4. I promise that if I break any of these promises, I'll sit down and re-read this contract.

5. I promise to remember why I'm trying to lose weight, especially when I'm tempted to eat something unhealthy, skip an exercise session or just give up.

6. I promise not to let outside influences - friends, family or lack of time - interfere with my determination to achieve my goal.

7. I promise not to let negative thoughts stop me from achieving my goal.

8. I promise to celebrate in style once I hit my target weight.

9. ....
....

10. ....
....

11. ....
....

12. ....
....

Signed: ....

Date & Place: ....

THE MUMMYLICIOUS
RECIPES

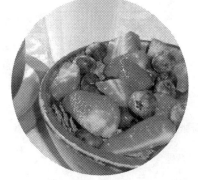

BREAKFAST RECIPE

RAISIN BRAN CEREAL WITH LOW-FAT MILK AND MIXED BERRIES

Ingredients: (serves 1)

1 serving (1 cup) of cereal

(whole-grain, containing bran or other high-fibre cereal)

1 cup of low fat milk

A handful of mixed berries (blueberries, strawberries, raspberries)

Instructions:

Pour cereal, berries and milk into a bowl.

Nutrient Information Per Serving:

Calories 360, Total Carbohydrates 75.3g, Dietary Fiber 12.8g,

Total Fat 4.0g. Vitamin A 27% • Vitamin C 50% • Calcium 34% • Iron 64%.

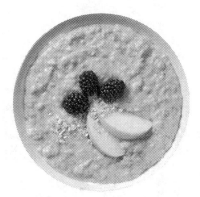

BREAKFAST RECIPE

HOT OATMEAL WITH LOW-FAT MILK AND MIXED FRUIT

Ingredients: (serves 1)

1 packet (45g) of plain instant oatmeal

2/3 cup of water

1 teaspoon of brown sugar (optional)

1/4 cup dried raisins or berries

1 cup of diced apples or kiwis

1 cup of low fat milk

A sprinkle of cinnamon powder (optional)

Instructions:

Mix oatmeal and water, and heat up in a microwave or on the stove. Place mixture in a bowl and add the dried raisins, diced apples, sugar (optional) and milk. You may also sprinkle a dash of cinnamon powder.

Nutrient Information Per Serving:

Calories 450, Total Carbohydrates 89.5g, Dietary Fiber 8.5g, Total Fat 5.7g. Vitamin A 11% • Vitamin C 10% • Calcium 35% • Iron 16%.

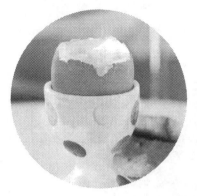

BREAKFAST RECIPE
SOFT BOILED EGG AND WHOLE-WHEAT TOAST

Ingredients: (serves 1)
1 egg
2 slices of whole-wheat bread, toasted
1/2 teaspoon (per slice of bread) of butter, margarine or a light spread of
your choice

Instructions:
Place the raw egg in a saucepan, add water (until 1 inch above the egg),
and cook over medium heat until the water begins to boil. Reduce the
heat to low and simmer for 2 to 3 minutes. Remove the egg with a spoon
or ladle and let it cool. Toast bread to your liking (add a thin layer of your
choice of spread) and serve with the soft boiled egg.

Nutrient Information Per Serving:
Calories 250, Total Carbohydrates 23.5g, Dietary Fiber 6.5g, Total Fat 8.2g.
Vitamin A 5% • Vitamin C 0% • Calcium 8% • Iron 12%

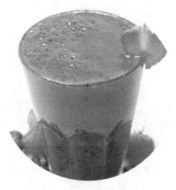

BREAKFAST RECIPE
WILD BERRY SMOOTHIE

Ingredients: (serves 1)
1 1/2 cups of unsweetened apple juice
1/2 cup of strawberries
1/2 cup of blueberries
1 banana

Instructions:
Pour juice into a blender and add the fruit. Process until smooth.

Nutrient Information Per Serving:
Calories 344, Total Carbohydrates 86.4g, Dietary Fiber 6.6g, Total Fat 1.3g.
Vitamin A 3% • Vitamin C 357% • Calcium 5% • Iron 12%.

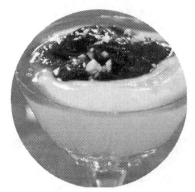

BREAKFAST RECIPE
STEWED PRUNES WITH LOW-FAT PLAIN YOGURT

Ingredients: (serves 1)
8-10 stewed prunes, pitted
2/3 cup of low-fat plain yogurt
1 tablespoon of honey (optional)

Instructions:
Place prunes and yogurt into a bowl, then drizzle with honey (optional).

Nutrient Information Per Serving:
Calories 284, Total Carbohydrates 68.2g, Dietary Fiber 5.1g, Total Fat 2.0g.
Vitamin A 2% • Vitamin C 2% • Calcium 30% • Iron 1%.

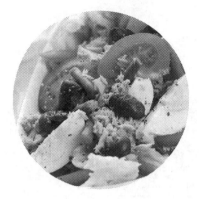

TUNA NIÇOISE SALAD

Ingredients: (serves 4)

1 1/2 cups of canned tuna

4 plum tomatoes, roughly chopped

115g extra fine French beans, cooked and drained

4 little gem lettuce hearts, quartered lengthways

1 red onion, finely sliced

4 eggs, cooked for 6 minutes in boiling water, peeled and halved

16 pitted black olives in brine

2 tablespoons of capers

Vinaigrette :

1 teaspoon of Dijon mustard

3 tablespoons of red wine vinegar

2 tablespoons of chopped fresh flat-leaf parsley

2 tablespoons of minced fresh tarragon

1/2 cup extra-virgin olive oil

Salt and freshly-ground black pepper, to taste

Instructions:

Make the dressing by whisking together the vinaigrette ingredients in a mixing bowl. Now assemble the salad. Place beans, olives, lettuce, red onions, tomatoes in a large mixing bowl. Pour on some vinaigrette and use tongs to toss the ingredients to coat well. Divide salad into serving bowls. Top with tuna, eggs, olives, cappers and serve.

Nutrient Information Per Serving:

Calories 450, Total Carbohydrates 28.5g, Dietary Fiber 10.8g, Total Fat 28g. Vitamin A 39% • Vitamin C 41% • Calcium 14% • Iron 23%.

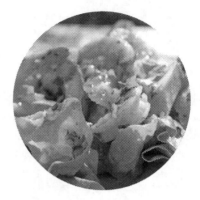

LUNCH RECIPE

THAI AVOCADO, PRAWNS AND POMELO SALAD

Ingredients: (serves 4)

1 packet of salad of your choice

1/2 cup of fresh mint

1/2 cup of fresh coriander

2 avocados, peeled, pit removed and sliced

1 large pomelo, peeled and segmented

200g of cooked, peeled prawns

Vinaigrette :

1/4 cup of lime juice

2 tablespoons of fish sauce

2 tablespoons of honey

2 tablespoons of sweet chili sauce

Salt and freshly-ground black pepper, to taste

Instructions:

Combine the salad, mint and coriander and arrange the avocados, pomelo segments and prawns over the leaves. Combine all the vinaigrette ingredients and mix well. Taste and adjust seasoning to achieve a sweet and sour, to slightly salty taste. Drizzle over the salad, season with salt and pepper and serve immediately.

Nutrient Information Per Serving:

Calories 317, Total Carbohydrates 34.3g, Dietary Fiber 8.8g, Total Fat 15.5g. Vitamin A 43% • Vitamin C 237% • Calcium 7% • Iron 22%.

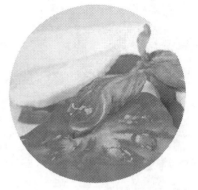

LUNCH RECIPE
TOMATOES, MOZZARELLA CHEESE AND FRESH BASIL SALAD

Ingredients: (serves 4)

2 heirloom tomatoes or 4 regular tomatoes, sliced

1 cup of fresh basil leaves

250g of fresh mozzarella cheese, sliced

1/4 cup extra virgin olive oil

3 tablespoons of balsamic wine vinegar

Salt and freshly-ground black pepper, to taste

Instructions:

In a circular design around the side of a plate, alternate fresh mozzarella slices with sliced tomatoes, overlapping for effect. Tear fresh basil leaves and sprinkle liberally over the slices. Add salt and freshly ground pepper to taste. Just before serving, drizzle on some top-quality extra-virgin olive oil and a touch of balsamic wine vinegar.

Nutrient Information Per Serving:

Calories 322, Total Carbohydrates 9.4g, Dietary Fiber 1.6g, Total Fat 25.1g. Vitamin A 33% • Vitamin C 28% • Calcium 44% • Iron 4%.

CRISPY CAESAR WITH GRILLED CHICKEN

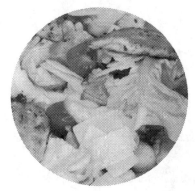

Ingredients: (serves 4)
400g of boneless skinless chicken breast halves
1/2 cup extra-virgin olive oil
3 tablespoons of fresh lemon juice
2 tablespoons of anchovy paste
2 cloves of garlic, minced
6 cups of torn romaine lettuce leaves
4 plum tomatoes, quartered
1/4 cup of grated or finely sliced Parmesan cheese
Salt and freshly-ground black pepper, to taste

Instructions:
Place chicken in large food storage bag. Combine oil, lemon juice, anchovy paste, garlic, salt and pepper in a small bowl. Reserve 1/3 cup of the marinade. Cover and refrigerate. Pour remaining marinade over the chicken in a bag. Seal the bag tightly, turning to coat. Marinate in the refrigerator at least 1 hour or for up to 4 hours, turning occasionally. Combine lettuce, tomatoes and cheese in a large bowl. Cover and refrigerate. If you don't have an outdoor grill, preheat your oven to 190°C and heat the grill pan on the top of the stove on high heat until it is smoking hot. Drain chicken, pouring marinade into a small saucepan. Bring marinade to a boil; boil for 1 minute. Put your chicken on the grill for 90 seconds per side. Do not overcook and do not move the chicken so you have those nice grill marks. Finish it up by putting the chicken into a pan with the rest of the boiled marinade and back into the oven for about 10-15 minutes at 100°C or until well cooked. Take the chicken out and let it rest for 5 minutes. Slice the warm chicken crosswise into 1/2 -inch-wide strips; add it to the lettuce, tomatoes and cheese mixture in the bowl, coat the chicken with the reserved 1/3-cup marinade which you have kept in the fridge (this serves as your vinaigrette), toss well and serve.

Nutrient Information Per Serving:
Calories 499, Total Carbohydrates 11.0g, Dietary Fiber 3.0g, Total Fat 19.4g. Vitamin A 124% • Vitamin C 80% • Calcium 33% • Iron 16%.

ROASTED PUMPKIN, BABY SPINACH, PINE NUTS AND RICOTTA CHEESE SALAD

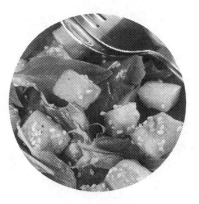

Ingredients: (serves 4)

600g of butternut pumpkin, deseeded, peeled and cut into wedges

250g of baby spinach leaves

40g of toasted pine nuts

100g of ricotta cheese (optional)

1 tablespoon of sesame seeds

Salt and freshly-ground black pepper, to taste

Vinaigrette :

2 teaspoons of honey

2 teaspoons of sesame seeds

1 tablespoon of fresh lemon juice

4 tablespoons of extra virgin olive oil

Instructions:

Preheat your oven to 220°C. Line a baking tray with non-stick baking paper. Place the pumpkin wedges in a large bowl. Drizzle with oil and honey. Season with salt and pepper. Gently toss until the pumpkin pieces are well coated. Place in a single layer on the lined tray. Bake, turning once during cooking, for 25 minutes or until golden brown. Remove from the oven and sprinkle evenly with the sesame seeds. Return to the oven and bake for another 5 minutes or until the seeds are lightly toasted. Remove from the oven and set aside for 30 minutes to cool. Combine the lemon juice, extra virgin olive oil and honey in a screw-top jar and shake until well combined. Season with salt and pepper. Place the pumpkin, spinach and pine nuts in a large bowl. Drizzle with the vinaigrette and gently toss. Serve topped with ricotta cheese.

Nutrient Information Per Serving:

Calories 322, Total Carbohydrates 9.4g, Dietary Fiber 1.6g, Total Fat 25.1g. Vitamin A 33% • Vitamin C 28% • Calcium 44% • Iron 4%.

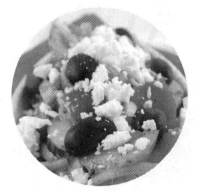

LUNCH RECIPE
CLASSIC GREEK SALAD

Ingredients: (serves 4)

4-5 large, ripe, tomatoes, cut into medium pieces or wedges

1 large red onion, chopped

1 cucumber, quartered lengthways, deseeded and chopped

1 green bell pepper, chopped

100g of feta cheese, sliced or crumbled

1/2 cup of chopped fresh oregano leaves

3 tablespoons of extra virgin olive oil

1 1/2 tablespoons of lemon juice

1 dozen Kalamata olives

Salt and freshly-ground black pepper, to taste

Instructions:

In a shallow salad bowl, combine tomatoes, cucumber and onion.
Sprinkle with salt and let sit for a few minutes so that the salt can draw
out the natural juices from the tomato and cucumber. Drizzle with olive
oil and sprinkle with oregano, and pepper to taste. Sprinkle feta cheese
and olives over salad and serve.

Nutrient Information Per Serving:

Calories 250, Total Carbohydrates 17.8g, Dietary Fiber 4.9g, Total Fat 17.6g.
Vitamin A 52% • Vitamin C 110% • Calcium 21% • Iron 14%.

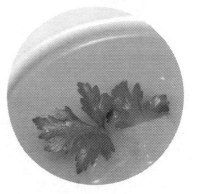

LUNCH RECIPE
PUMPKIN AND APPLE SOUP

Ingredients: (serves 4)

2 onions, peeled and chopped

1 clove of garlic, peeled and crushed

1 tablespoon of olive oil

500g of pumpkin, skinned, seeded and cubed

2 baking apples, peeled, cored and chopped

2 1/2 cups of vegetable stock

1 1/2 cups of unsweetened apple juice

2 sprigs of fresh parsley to garnish

Salt and freshly-ground black pepper, to taste

Instructions:

Heat the oil in a large saucepan and add the onions and the garlic. Cook for 2 minutes and then add the pumpkin, chopped apples and sage. Cook for another 2 minutes, season well and add the stock and apple juice. Bring to boil and simmer for 15-20 minutes until the ingredients are tender. Liquidise in a blender and serve hot.

Nutrient Information Per Serving:

Calories 221, Total Carbohydrates 46.6g, Dietary Fiber 8.6g, Total Fat 5.9g. Vitamin A 396% • Vitamin C 111% • Calcium 13% • Iron 22%.

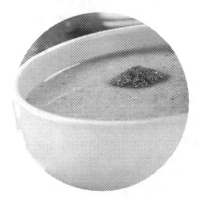

LUNCH RECIPE
BROCCOLI AND GOAT CHEESE SOUP

Ingredients: (serves 4)

2 tablespoons of butter

1 finely chopped onion

1 finely chopped celery stalk

3 cups of broth (chicken or vegetable)

8 cups of broccoli florets

3 tablespoons of butter

4 slices of soft goat cheese

Salt and freshly-ground black pepper, to taste

Instructions:

Melt the 2 tablespoons of butter in a pan. Add the finely chopped onions and celery and sauté until soft. Add the broccoli and the stock to the pan. Simmer for approximately 10 minutes until the broccoli is tender. Add the slices of goat cheese and stir until melted. Purée the soup in a blender and serve hot.

Nutrient Information Per Serving:

Calories 341, Total Carbohydrates 15.6g, Dietary Fiber 5.1g, Total Fat 25g. Vitamin A 40% • Vitamin C 265% • Calcium 33% • Iron 12%.

LUNCH RECIPE
WILD MUSHROOM SOUP WITH LIGHT CRÈME

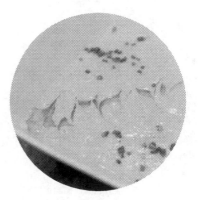

Ingredients: (serves 4)

500g of mixed wild mushrooms

50g of butter

1 onion, chopped

1 clove of garlic, crushed

1 thyme sprig

3 1/2 cups of vegetable stock

5 tablespoons of light crème fraîche (or if you prefer, light sour cream)

Finely chopped chives to garnish

1 teaspoon of truffle oil (optional)

Salt and freshly-ground black pepper, to taste

Instructions:

Heat half the butter in a saucepan, then gently sizzle the onion, garlic and thyme for 5 minutes until softened and starting to brown. Add the mixed wild mushrooms. Leave to cook for 5 minutes or until they go limp. Pour over the stock and bring to a boil, then simmer for 20 minutes. Stir in the light crème fraîche, then simmer for a few minutes more. Purée the soup in a blender, pass through a sifter, scatter over the chives and add a drizzle of truffle oil, then serve hot.

Nutrient Information Per Serving:

Calories 250, Total Carbohydrates 9.9g, Dietary Fiber 2.2g, Total Fat 21.1g. Vitamin A 7% • Vitamin C 12% • Calcium 2% • Iron 5%.

93

CHILLED GAZPACHO WITH CREAMY AVOCADO SOUP

Ingredients: (serves 4)

1 cucumber, peeled, seeded, and finely diced

1 big red pepper, seeded and finely diced

3 celery stalks, finely diced

1 ripe avocado, halved, and pit removed

Juice of 1 lemon

4 tablespoons of olive oil

1 clove of garlic, finely chopped

1/2 cup of water or crushed ice

Chive sprigs to garnish

Salt and freshly-ground black pepper, to taste

Instructions:

Combine all ingredients and diced vegetables in a blender. Process until smooth. Add water or crushed ice depending on the thickness of the soup you want. Chill and serve in soup bowls, garnished with chive sprigs or diced cucumbers, if desired.

Nutrient Information Per Serving:

Calories 237, Total Carbohydrates 14.0g, Dietary Fiber 4.8g, Total Fat 21.1g. Vitamin A 23% • Vitamin C 117% • Calcium 3% • Iron 4%.

DINNER RECIPE

HONEY MUSTARD GLAZED SALMON FILLETS AND STEAMED FRENCH BEANS

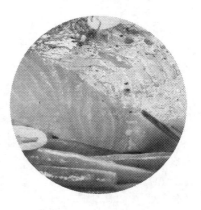

Ingredients: (serves 4)

4 (140g) salmon fillets

2 tablespoons of fresh lemon juice

2 tablespoons of Dijon mustard

2 tablespoons of honey

1 teaspoon of finely grated lemon zest

400 grams of French beans (ends removed)

Flat parsley to garnish

Salt and freshly-ground black pepper, to taste

Instructions:

In a shallow baking dish, combine lemon juice, Dijon, honey, and lemon zest. Stir together. Season both sides of the salmon fillets with salt and pepper and place in the baking dish (cover and marinate for 1 hour in the fridge). Flip salmon to coat in glaze. When ready to cook, preheat oven to 200°C. Bake 20 minutes or until fish is fork-tender and serve with a generous portion of steamed French beans and flat parsley to garnish. To steam French beans, place them in a microwave-safe bowl, add no more water than what it takes to rinse your vegetables before washing. Cover the bowl with a microwave safe plastic cover, leaving one corner open to vent. Microwave for 3 to 4 minutes.

Nutrient Information Per Serving:

Calories 426, Total Carbohydrates 13.7g, Dietary Fiber 2.4g, Total Fat 22.4g. Vitamin A 41% • Vitamin C 59% • Calcium 6% • Iron 24%.

APRICOT CHICKEN WITH FRESH THYME AND STEAMED BRUSSELS SPROUTS

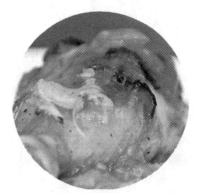

Ingredients: (serves 4)

6 chicken thigh fillets

2 x 45g of French onion soup mix

2 x 420g tins of apricot nectar (containing whole apricot pieces)

1 cup of flour to coat the chicken

Fresh thyme sprigs

3 tablespoons of olive oil

450g of Brussels sprouts

Salt and freshly-ground black pepper, to taste

Instructions:

Preheat oven to 180°C. Place flour, salt and pepper in a shallow dish. Lightly coat chicken pieces in seasoned flour, shaking off excess. Heat the olive oil in a deep, large, heavy-based frying pan over medium heat. Cook chicken, in batches, for 2 to 3 minutes each side or until golden. Place chicken in a baking or casserole dish. In a large jug combine the French onion soup packets and apricot nectar, mix well and pour over chicken. Cover and bake at 180°C for two hours. Garnish with fresh thyme and serve with steamed Brussels sprouts (Brussels sprouts takes approximately 7 minutes in the microwave).

Nutrient Information Per Serving:

Calories 465, Total Carbohydrates 54.5g, Dietary Fiber 6.1g, Total Fat 17.1g. Vitamin A 72% • Vitamin C 350% • Calcium 7% • Iron 24%.

BEEF BOURGUIGNON WITH PEARL ONIONS AND MUSHROOMS, SERVED WITH STEAMED CARROTS

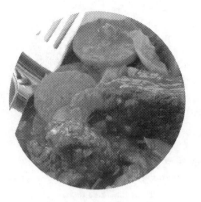

Ingredients: (serves 4)
500g of beef shoulder or beef cheek (stewing beef), cut in two-inch cubes
1 onion, peeled and chopped
2 cups of button mushrooms, cut in halves
2 celery stalks, chopped
3 cups of red wine
2 cups of beef stock
1/2 cup of flour
2 tablespoons of olive oil
Flat parsley to garnish
Fresh thyme sprigs
1 clove of garlic, mashed
12 small white pearl onions, peeled
400g of carrots sliced into rounds
Salt and freshly-ground black pepper, to taste

Instructions:
Preheat oven to 130°C. Place flour, salt and pepper in a shallow dish. Lightly coat beef cube pieces in seasoned flour, shaking off excess. Heat 2 tablespoons of olive oil in a deep, large, heavy-based frying pan over medium heat and once hot, add the beef cubes. Cook until brown. Remove the beef and set aside. In the same pan, cook the chopped onions and celery for 2 or 3 minutes, then return the beef to the pan. Add salt and pepper. Cook for an additional 3 or 4 minutes. Pour in the red wine and enough bouillon to cover all the ingredients. Add the garlic, mushrooms, pearl onions and fresh herbs. Bring to a boil. Cover the pan and place in the heated oven. Cook at 130°C for 3 hours. The beef will be ready when it is fork-tender. Serve beef with some sauce, mushrooms and pearl onions, and garnish with parsley, thyme and with a generous serving of steamed carrots (carrots take approximately 5 minutes in the microwave).

Nutrient Information Per Serving:
Calories 650, Total Carbohydrates 39.5g, Dietary Fiber 8.2g, Total Fat 25.8g. Vitamin A 356% • Vitamin C 47% • Calcium 20% • Iron 80%.

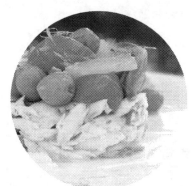

DINNER RECIPE
OVEN-COOKED SEA BASS STUFFED WITH FENNEL AND LEMON, SERVED WITH ROASTED OLIVES AND TOMATOES

Ingredients: (serves 4)

4 medium sized sea bass fish, cleaned, scaled and ready to cook

2 fennel bulbs, cut in long slices

3 fresh lemons, cut in wedges

Fresh tarragon

1 clove of garlic, crushed

2 cups of green olives, pitted

3 cups of cherry tomatoes

3 tablespoons of olive oil

Salt and freshly-ground black pepper, to taste

Instructions:

Preheat your oven to 180°C . Stuff your fish with lemon wedges, fennel slices, olive oil, fresh tarragon, salt and pepper and place on an oven tray on aluminum foil. Arrange the olives and cherry tomatoes around the fish in the same tray. Cook for 25-30 minutes at 180°C. Serve garnished with fresh tarragon, a dash of olive oil and the lemon, olives, cherry tomatoes and fennel which have cooked with the fish. You can use a stacking cylinder for a nicer presentation.

Nutrient Information Per Serving:

Calories 376, Total Carbohydrates 19.5g, Dietary Fiber 7.1g, Total Fat 17.4g. Vitamin A 17% • Vitamin C 119% • Calcium 20% • Iron 13%.

DINNER RECIPE

SEAFOOD BAKE SERVED WITH A CRISPY GREEN SALAD

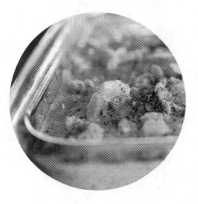

Ingredients: (serves 4)
4 pieces of cod or salmon fillets
300g of prawns, out of their shell
2 cups of fresh low fat milk
3 bay leaves
500g of broccoli, chopped in small chunks
1 cup of grated low fat cheddar cheese
3 tablespoons of flour
3 tablespoons of butter
1 1/2 cups of fresh low fat milk
Green salad and vinaigrette of your choice
Salt and freshly-ground black pepper, to taste

Instructions:

Pre-heat your oven to 180°C. Steam or microwave your broccoli for 3-4 minutes and set aside. In another pan, boil peeled prawns in water for about 5 minutes or less, depending on the size of the prawns. Once their flesh turns white and they start to float, you can take them out of the water.

In a third pan, boil the fish fillets in milk with the bay leaves, on low fire until cooked (approximately 35 minutes depending on the thickness of your fish fillets). Take the fillets out of the milk and set them aside to cool. In a baking dish, place broccoli pieces, followed by fish flakes and prawns on top of each other.

Now prepare your white sauce: In a small pan, melt the butter at low fire and add the flour mixture then the milk and mix until mixture thickens; season with salt and pepper. Pour the white sauce to coat the prawns, fish and broccoli. Sprinkle with grated cheddar cheese and cook 30 minutes at 180°C and until the top is golden brown. Serve with a crispy green salad and vinaigrette of your choice.

Nutrient Information Per Serving:

Calories 516, Total Carbohydrates 42.5g, Dietary Fiber 5.4g, Total Fat 20.3g.
Vitamin A 55% • Vitamin C 237% • Calcium 35% • Iron 31%.

DINNER RECIPE

CHICKEN SATAY WITH PEANUT SAUCE AND ROASTED RED PEPPERS

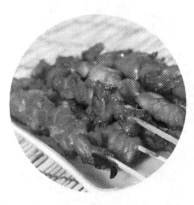

Ingredients: (serves 4)

500 g of chicken breast meat, (cut into
5mm thick, 2.5cm wide strips)
5 red peppers
1 cup of fresh coriander leaves
Salt and freshly-ground black pepper, to taste

Peanut sauce:

2 tablespoons of smooth peanut butter
200ml of coconut cream
2 teaspoons of red Thai curry paste
1 tablespoon of fish sauce
1 tablespoon of soft light brown sugar
Salt and freshly-ground black pepper, to taste

Marinade:

2 tablespoons of vegetable oil
2 tablespoons of soy sauce
2 tablespoons of tamarind paste
1 lemon-grass stalk (tender inner part only), chopped roughly
2 garlic cloves, crushed
1 teaspoon of ground cumin
1 teaspoon of ground coriander
1 tablespoon of lime juice
1 tablespoon of soft light brown sugar

Instructions:

Thread the chicken onto bamboo skewers and transfer to a rectangular dish. Add the marinade to the chicken and toss to coat. Cover with cling film and refrigerate for at least 1 hour. Grill the chicken on a barbecue or under an oven grill for 3-5 minutes at 180°C on each side, or until the chicken is cooked through and serve with peanut sauce, roasted red peppers and fresh coriander.

To make marinade:

Place the oil, soy sauce, tamarind paste, lemon grass, garlic, cumin, coriander, lime juice and sugar in a food processor and blend to make a paste.

To roast your peppers:

Place clean whole fresh peppers on a baking dish. Broil under medium heat, 180°C, turning frequently, as necessary, until the entire pepper skin has turned black and blistery. Remove from oven and place peppers into an airtight container with a lid. Let the peppers rest in the container for 10 to 15 minutes to build up steam that is needed to aid in the removal of the skin. Remove from container and peel off the skin. Cut the pepper in half, core and remove seeds. Slice peppers into strips and serve with the chicken satay sticks.

To make peanut sauce:

Put the peanut butter, coconut cream, red Thai curry paste, fish sauce and sugar in a pan. Heat gently, stirring, to form a smooth sauce.

Nutrient Information Per Serving:

Calories 503, Total Carbohydrates 24.6g, Dietary Fiber 1.5g, Total Fat 20.45g. Vitamin A 10% • Vitamin C 112% • Calcium 6% • Iron 24%.

PRAWNS COOKED IN COCONUT MILK AND LIME JUICE, SERVED WITH STEAMED GREEN ASPARAGUS

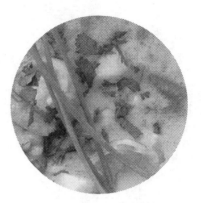

Ingredients: (serves 4)

500g of prawns out of their shell

6 tomatoes, peeled and sliced

1 fresh ginger root, sliced in very thin strips

1 cup of fresh coriander, finely chopped

200ml of coconut milk

2 cloves of garlic, finely chopped

Juice of 5 limes

1 onion, chopped

2 tablespoons of olive oil

16-20 stalks of green-asparagus

Salt and freshly-ground black pepper, to taste

Instructions:

Marinate the prawns in the lime juice, fresh ginger, fresh coriander and garlic for at least 1 hour in the fridge.

Separate the marinade from the prawns. Pass the rest of the marinade through a sieve, and keep the ginger, garlic and herbs, but discard the juice. Heat the olive oil in a pan or casserole dish. Sauté the garlic, ginger and herbs from the marinade; add the chopped onion and cook until soft. Add in the prawns as well as the tomatoes and cook till the prawns change colour. Add in the coconut milk and cover. Simmer for at least 20 minutes. Serve garnished with fresh coriander and with steamed asparagus (asparagus take approximately 4 to 6 minutes in the microwave).

Nutrient Information Per Serving:

Calories 599, Total Carbohydrates 49.2g, Dietary Fiber 16.4g, Total Fat 15.7g. Vitamin A 42% • Vitamin C 69% • Calcium 18% • Iron 38%.

CHICKEN CROQUETTES WITH A CAULIFLOWER GRATIN

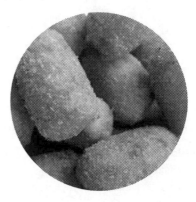

Ingredients: (serves 4-6)
For chicken croquettes:
6 chicken thighs
4 spring onions, finely chopped
1 egg
1 small onion, finely chopped
1 cup of bread crumbs
1 chicken Knorr cube, crushed
3 tablespoons of olive oil
Salt and freshly-ground black pepper, to taste

For cauliflower bake:
1 whole cauliflower cut in small pieces
1 cup of grated low fat cheddar cheese
3 tablespoons of flour
3 tablespoons of butter
1 1/2 cups of fresh low fat milk

Instructions:
Chicken Croquettes: Boil the chicken thighs in water, with the chopped onion and some salt and pepper for about 1 hour at low fire. Take out the chicken pieces and let them cool. Discard water and onion. Separate the chicken flesh from the bone and chop finely. Add the chopped spring onions, and the Knorr chicken powder and mix thoroughly. Now form the mixture into small rolls and set aside. Dredge the rolls in the beaten egg mixture and coat with bread crumbs. Lightly pan fry in olive oil until breadcrumbs turn brown on both sides (approximately 2 minutes).

Cauliflower Bake: Pre-heat your oven to 180°C. Steam or microwave cauliflower for 5-7 minutes. Now prepare white sauce: In a small pan, melt the butter at low fire and add the flour mixture then the milk and mix until mixture thickens; season with salt and pepper. Place the cauliflower pieces in a baking dish. Pour the white sauce over and sprinkle with grated cheddar cheese. Bake for 30 minutes at 180°C and until golden brown. Serve with chicken croquettes.

Nutrient Information Per Serving :
Calories 585, Total Carbohydrates 35.3g, Dietary Fiber 6.0g, Total Fat 28.0g. Vitamin A 13% • Vitamin C 136% • Calcium 30% • Iron 22%.

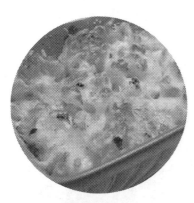

DINNER RECIPE

STUFFED BELL PEPPERS WITH GROUND BEEF, CORN AND ZUCCHINI, SERVED WITH A CRISPY GREEN SALAD

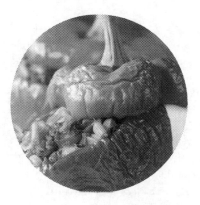

Ingredients: (serves 4)

400g of minced beef

1 cup whole kernel corn

1 medium-sized zucchini, cut and chopped into very small cubes

4 large bell peppers, any colour (red, orange, green, yellow)

175g of tomato paste

1 small onion, finely chopped

2 cloves of garlic, finely chopped

2 tablespoons of olive oil

Green salad and vinaigrette of your choice

Salt and freshly-ground black pepper, to taste

Instructions:

Pre-heat your oven to 160°C. Now prepare bell peppers by cutting off the tops and removing all the seeds. Keep the peppers and their tops and set aside. In a large pan, heat olive oil and sauté the onions until soft, then add the garlic and minced beef. Cook, while stirring, until brown. Add the chopped zucchinis and stir then 5 minutes later add the corn and the tomato paste, salt and pepper and cover for 5 minutes. Gently stuff the peppers with the ground beef and vegetable mixture and place them in a baking dish. Cook in the oven for 2 hours at 160°C and serve with a crispy green salad and vinaigrette of your choice.

Nutrient Information Per Serving :

Calories 457, Total Carbohydrates 28.2g, Dietary Fiber 6.4g, Total Fat 20.9g. Vitamin A 95% • Vitamin C 293% • Calcium 7% • Iron 32%.

DINNER RECIPE
ROASTED LEG OF LAMB SERVED WITH
FLAGEOLET BEANS AND ROASTED TOMATOES

Ingredients: (serves 4-6)

1 leg of lamb

4 sprigs of rosemary

4 cloves of garlic, crushed

1 cup of Madeira wine

1 cup of water

6 medium tomatoes, cut in halves

2 x 400g tins of flageolet beans

Flat parsley to garnish

Salt and freshly-ground black pepper, to taste

Instructions:

Pre-heat your oven to 200°C. Place lamb in a roasting pan, massage with garlic and sprinkle with rosemary, salt and pepper. Cook for 35 minutes at 200°C. Take out, and pour the Madeira wine and water over the lamb. Add the tomatoes around the lamb and return to the oven and cook for an additional 35 minutes. Take the leg of lamb out and let it rest for 10 minutes on a wooden board covered in aluminum foil. Put one more cup of water in the cooking pan and mix with the cooking juices. Pour gravy through a sifter and spoon out as much oil and fat as possible.

In a medium pan, pour flageolet beans straight from the tin, heat up and bring to a light boil for approximately 10 minutes.

Slice the meat and drizzle with some of the gravy. Serve with the flageolet beans and tomatoes and garnish with flat parsley .

Nutrient Information Per Serving :

Calories 628, Total Carbohydrates 23.5g, Dietary Fiber 5.6g, Total Fat 29.0g. Vitamin A 24% • Vitamin C 45% • Calcium 12% • Iron 46%.

ACKNOWLEDGMENTS

Like so many authors before me, I've had days when I've felt like giving up, deleting everything I've written so far and simply forgetting about this whole book project altogether. Sometimes I would say to myself: "Why go on? It sounds terrible! Who is going to want to read this anyway?" But a few people, who believed in me, kept me going and gave me the courage to surmount my self-doubt and finish this book.

Straight at number one, my darling husband Steven, who is my best friend and partner in life, you have my deepest gratitude for always believing in me. For the countless hours you've spent listening to me reading back my various chapters, for helping me find the title of my book, for constantly trying to put yourself into the mind (and body) of a post-pregnancy mum, for always giving me your honest opinion and for taking the picture of my book's back cover (when Angeline and I were not even looking), you deserve a medal in addition to all my love and devotion.

To my Mum, who is the woman I love and admire the most in the world, thank you for your time and patience while reading all my drafts and for listening to me yak away about my various ideas for the next few chapters of the book. You've been by my side the first few months after all four births, and your presence during those important moments of my life meant more to me than you can ever imagine.

Furthermore, when I think back about when I really started enjoying writing, and about how I found the courage and desire to embark on the project of putting together a book, my first thought goes to my extremely talented editor and girlfriend, Giselle Go, former editor of Harper's Bazaar Magazine Singapore and current editor in chief at Mediacorp. Giselle, you ignited in me the passion for the written word, by giving me a chance to contribute articles to Bazaar and for this, I am forever grateful. Thank you for your belief in me, for your support, and for giving me this opportunity to begin with.

To my dear family friend and other editor, Bonnie Melvin, who writes fiction and works at the International Herald Tribune in Paris, we've known each other for many years and throughout you have been incredibly kind, generous and supportive of me. Thank you for your patience, extreme attention to detail and for spending so many hours combing through my manuscript. I could not have published this book without your help and guidance.

To my talented illustrator, Wearn, thank you for your beautiful and entertaining watercolour drawings. You've really made my book come alive and it has truly been a pleasure working with you on this project.

To my sister, Nathalie, I value and respect your opinion immensely. What you say in a few words always resonates with me. You have a way of continuously being spot-on with your observations and recommendations. Thank you for your advice, and for designing this wonderful book layout as well as my book's website, and most importantly, thank you for your support always.

To my brother, Guillaume, who is probably as health and fitness obsessed as I am, I loved getting your input and well-researched ideas on nutrition and diet. Thank you for your backing and encouragement and for always making me laugh with your crazy antics.

To my darling sisters-in-law, Donna and Vesna, and to my beloved niece-in-law Kirsty, thank you for taking the time to read my drafts and for your wonderful advice and suggestions. You have been so kind, loving and thoughtful over the years, and that has always meant the world to me.

To my closest friends, Mike, Anjali, Yumi, Trina and Kiwha, thank you for giving me your honest feedback, comments and ideas on my first chapter and initial document. Your impressions, without a doubt, helped me shape the direction and tone of my manuscript thereafter.

To my dearest and most treasured friend, Kristin, the book would not have been the same without your contribution along the way. For your insightful comments, creative suggestions, fun insights and for writing the foreword of my book, you have my deepest gratitude and sincere recognition.

And finally, my biggest thank you goes to my four children. You are the light of my life and the reason this book exists. Words cannot express how much happiness you give me everyday. Thank you for your unconditional love and for making me a better person.

ABOUT THE AUTHOR

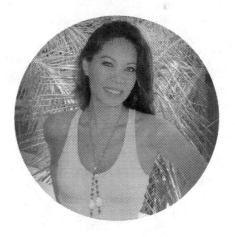

Of French and Filipino descent, Christine Amour-Levar is a freelance writer, sports editor and marketing consultant currently based in Singapore, where she lives with her husband and four children. She grew up between Manila, Paris and Tokyo, and has travelled extensively due to her many work commitments. Christine's career started in Japan in advertising, where after graduating Cum Laude from Sophia University in Tokyo, with a BA in Business and Economics and a minor in Japanese language, she joined the firm of McCann-Erickson as an account executive. Her experience in advertising, her language skills (she speaks six languages: French, English, Spanish, Japanese, Tagalog and conversational Portuguese) and her passion for sports, consequently led her to work in marketing for Nike in the United States, Latin America, France and Singapore.

Christine also holds a degree from the New York School of Interior Design and worked briefly for Philippe Stack in Paris, before rejoining Nike and moving to Singapore in 2005. After her stint running the marketing department for Nike Singapore from 2005 to 2007, she saw a gap in the retail market for Brazilian fashion, which persuaded her to launch Singapore's first and only Brazilian multi-brand fashion boutique, Beijaflor. Christine then successfully sold her business in 2010, and currently contributes articles to various regional publications such as Harper's Bazaar Magazine Singapore, while also working as a marketing consultant with the Special Olympics Asia Pacific regional office.

SOURCES CONSULTED

Women's Healthcare topics, "Causes, Prevention and Treatment of Pregnancy Stretch Marks":
www.womenshealthcaretopics.com/stretch_mark_treatment.htm

Breastfeeding.com, "The Secrets of Breastfeeding and Weight Loss ":
www.breastfeeding.com/all_about/all_about_lose_weight.html

Wikipedia, "Linea Nigra":
http://en.wikipedia.org/wiki/Linea_nigra

La Leche League International, "How Can I Lose Weight Safely While Breastfeeding?":
www.llli.org/faq/diet.html

Breastfeeding Basics, "Nutrition, Exercise, and Weight Loss While Breastfeeding":
www.breastfeedingbasics.com/html/Nutrition.shtml

Pregnancyinfo.net, "Getting Back into Shape After Baby":
www.pregnancy-info.net/postbody.html

Public Health Grey Bruce Unit, "Breast and Nipple Care":
www.publichealthgreybruce.on.ca/family/breastfeeding/BreastNippleCare.htm
Australian Breastfeeding Association, "Weaning":
www.breastfeeding.asn.au/bfinfo/weaning.html

Livestrong, Partners of the Lance Armstrong Foundation, "The Best Way to Breath While Exercising":
www.livestrong.com/article/367871-the-best-way-to-breathe-while-exercising/

Silverston Consulting, "How to Strengthen Your Resolve", by Robert Silverston:
www.robertsilverstone.com/articles/How%20to%20Strengthen%20Your%20Resolve.pdf

Psychology @ Suite101, "Setting Yourself Up for Success":
www.suite101.com/content/visualization-a17777#ixzz1EkkadimB

Mayo Clinic, "Low-carb diet: Can it help you lose weight?":
www.mayoclinic.com/health/low-carb-diet/NU00279

Associated Content, "High-Fiber Breakfast Choices":
www.associatedcontent.com/article/565505/highfiber_breakfast_choices.html?cat=5

Livestrong, Partners of the Lance Armstrong Foundation, "Snacks for Dieting": www.livestrong.com/snacks-for-dieting/

Mayo Clinic, "Ways to enjoy more whole grains" and "Whole grains vs. refined grains":
www.mayoclinic.com/health/whole-grains/NU00204

Mayo Clinic, "Cellulite":
www.mayoclinic.com/health/cellulite/DS00891

Medicinenet.com, "Endorphins: Natural Pain and Stress Fighters":
www.medicinenet.com/script/main/art.asp?articlekey=55001

Today's Women and Health, "Benefits of Pilates":
www.todays-women-and-health.com/benefits-of-pilates.html